DEAR MENOPAUSE, I DO NOT FEAR YOU!

A Modern Woman's Guide To Thriving Through Midlife

SOMA MANDAL, M.D.

© 2019 Dr. Soma Mandal

All rights reserved. No part of this publication may be reproduced, stored in a retrieval system, or transmitted in any form or by any means – electronic, mechanical, photocopy, recording, or any other – except for brief quotations in printed reviews or articles, without the prior written permission of the publisher.

Published by Premier Physician Media

Cover and Book Design by Premier Physician Marketing

Printed in the United States of America

ISBN: 9781692335564

"I see menopause as the start of the next fabulous phase of life as a woman. Now is a time to "tune in" to our bodies and embrace this new chapter. If anything, I feel more myself and love my body more now, at 58 years old, than ever before."

KIM CATTRALL, ACTOR

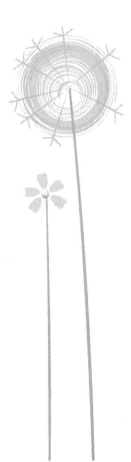

This book is dedicated to my husband, Suneel, who is the best thing that has happened to me, and also to the many friends, colleagues and mentors who have helped me along the way.

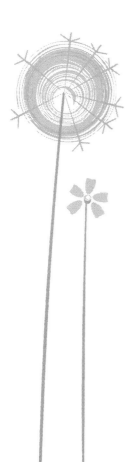

TABLE OF CONTENTS

	Introduction	1
1.	Meno-WHAT? Just What Is Going On With My Brain, Body And…	5
2.	Menopause Myth Busting	13
3.	Am I In Menopause Or…	23
4.	But My Body Never Used To Look Like This!	29
5.	Sprouting Silver – How To Deal With Gray Hair, Hair Loss And Changes To Our Scalp	37
6.	Clearing The Brain Fog	43
7.	Breast Talk	49
8.	Heart Health	55
9.	Taming The Thyroid & Menopause Madness	61
10.	Getting Your Skin Glow On	67
11.	Reclaiming Your Goddess	71
12.	Night Sweats, Hot Flashes	79
13.	Building Strong Bones	87
14.	Hormone Therapy Demystified (And Why It's Not Right For Everyone)	93

15. When East Meets West: Using Natural Therapies	**99**
16. Meditation, Yoga, Pilates And Other Ways To Transform Body & Spirit	**105**
17. Let's Talk Supplements	**111**
18. Menopause Meets Culture	**117**
19. Menopause For Women Of Color	**121**
Conclusion	**125**
About Dr. Soma Mandal	**127**
Get In Touch With Dr. Soma Mandal	**128**
References	**129**

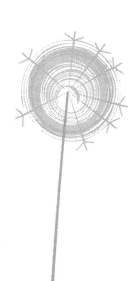

INTRODUCTION

*"You are more powerful than you know;
you are beautiful just as you are."*
MELISSA ETHERIDGE

There is probably no other word that carries more meaning and more mystique for women than the word *menopause*. It is the word that we all somehow come to know as young girls and then worry about as we get older. And, what we knew as girls, we often come to find out isn't exactly what happens at all. Sometimes we're relieved!

Depending on where and how you grew up, you may have formed ideas and notions about menopause that were either very cliché or even completely inaccurate. You may have been fortunate to have strong female role models from whom you were able to learn about what would come. It's probably safe to say that most of us probably entered our adult years with a blend of fact, fiction, advice from "Dr. Google" and a healthy dose of apprehension.

We can probably all point to someone that we knew as a child who was "going through the change" and the whispered comments, knowing glances and sometimes even absence of that person at family events. The women surrounding her "knew." The men in her life were left scratching their heads wondering what happened to that sweet lady they married!

Why is it that we do such a great job at educating our girls about what to expect during puberty, and that roller-coaster ride of pregnancy and becoming a mother – but when it comes to talking about menopause the conversation just stops? It's just a black hole that women who are forty plus fall into and are left on their own to find their way out of.

Thankfully, things are changing.

If you've started your menopause journey, or suspect you might have – or just want to know what lies ahead – bravo! Menopause is not something to fear or be ashamed of. It doesn't mean you have to trade in your skinny jeans for elasticized sweat pants, or that you're going to feel cranky, sweaty, or foggy-headed, for the rest of your life. Perhaps most importantly, menopause doesn't mean that you won't feel like yourself ever again. If managed properly, it can mean the exact opposite – the rebirth of a better you! A happier you. A less-stressed you. And perhaps for the first time in your life, it can give you the permission you need to finally put your own needs ahead of everyone else's.

Menopause *really can* be the most fulfilling and empowering time in a woman's life.

And that's what this book is about.

In the following pages, you're going to learn about menopause in a whole new way. We'll take the mystery out of it, so you can be armed with facts. We'll explore just what is happening and what to expect as the process unfolds. And we'll talk about practical, real life strategies of dealing with the unique physical, emotional and social changes that come with this process.

But before we dive in, let me introduce myself!

I am a board-certified internist based in Berkeley Heights, New Jersey who specializes in midlife women's health and have helped thousands of women successfully navigate the menopause journey and reinvent themselves along their journey. I earned my MD at New York University School of Medicine and was lucky enough to win a prestigious research fellowship at Oxford University in England, although I have to confess that neither of my parents were keen on me becoming a doctor!

Four fun facts about me:

1. I met my husband through online dating (yes it really does work, be brave, go for it!).
2. My favorite vacation place is Yellowstone Park. There aren't many places in the world I would return to vacation to, but this is definitely one of them. Add it to your bucket list if you haven't been already!
3. I am the proud mother to a beautiful six-year-old girl, who keeps me on my toes and my head spinning as I run from piano recitals, to dance classes to … well, I'm sure you know how it goes.
4. I can knit and crochet up a storm – it's my way of relaxing and unwinding after a hectic day at the clinic.

INTRODUCTION

As a child I had a lot of medical issues – bad asthma and allergies. Back then there weren't a lot of treatment options, but I remember being dragged to the doctor's office a lot of the time, which strangely I really enjoyed. I felt comfortable there – the busy-ness of the clinic, the doctors and nurses in white coats hovering over me, asking lots of questions and doing their best to help me. I found it really comforting. Even though being an MD wasn't in my parents' grand plans for me, they did tell my sister and I over and over again that whatever we chose, we needed to help people.

That really struck a chord with me. I have always been interested in women's health – I watched my mother juggle working in a bank with raising two exuberant daughters and the toll that took on her health – especially as she got older. Now as a working mom who's perimenopausal (don't worry if you don't know what that means yet, it's explained in the next chapter), juggling a very full-time job along with husband and child – I have a whole new appreciation for her.

A darker side of my upbringing, which I believe also led me to my desire to help women and focus on women's health, is that I was sexually assaulted as a child by an acquaintance of the family. I thought I had dealt with those issues – that is until I got pregnant and had my own daughter and everything came back to the surface. It's hard for me to even talk about it, but as you're taking the time to read my book, I think it's important for me to talk about it with you. Just in case you've had something similar happen, or someone you love has. I've found that by shining a flashlight on these dark things, we take away their power over us, and we can start to heal – and help others in the process. Plus, if you've been through it also, it's something else big we share in common.

So enough with the introductions, let's get started, shall we! Like you, I'm on my own menopause journey, my own journey of maturing as a woman – we're in this together!

"It is so liberating to really know what I want, what truly makes me happy, what I will not tolerate. I have learned that it is no one else's job to take care of me but me."

BEYONCE

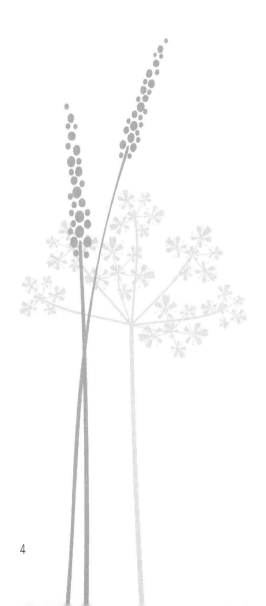

CHAPTER ONE

Meno-What? Just What Is Going On With My Brain, Body And..?

"A woman is the full circle. Within her is the power to create, nurture and transform."

Diane Mariechild

One morning, you wake up and something feels different. Something is not wrong but not quite right either. Hmm…

Maybe you start noticing little changes:

- My skin is a little drier than usual, kind of crepey in spots
- My hair just won't behave
- I can't remember anything lately
- My period late shows up late. It's very heavy. It's very light. It can't seem to make up it's mind. And sometimes it stays around longer than usual.
- The scale says what?!
- OMG was that just a hot flash??

What on earth is going on?

THE SIGNS OF THE TIME

The sense of "not quite the right" and the little changes you're seeing are signs that things are about to change. Those signs are telling you that your body is beginning the transition from your child-bearing years to post-childbearing, mature adulthood. Congratulations and welcome to the big "M." Like billions of women who have gone before us, you are about to join an elite group of women who are lucky enough to begin the process of menopause.

Lucky you say? Absolutely.

As a little girl, my Mom always told me that it was a privilege to age. Now that I'm going through perimenopause and have made it my life's work to help thousands of women successfully navigate their change, I really appreciate the wisdom of her words.

Contrary to popular belief and a few old wives tales, menopause doesn't come on suddenly. It doesn't come creeping like a thief in the night and silently steal your period. It is a process of the body preparing to cease its child-bearing functions. This process happens gradually over time. Sometimes that process is very subtle – barely noticeable – but for others the changes are front and center and very evident.

One thing is true for all women: all of us experience menopause, and it brings changes to us physically, emotionally and socially. We are a sisterhood united in growing older, and undergoing one more transformation – one more chrysalis to the most spectacular butterfly of all!

We all hear about "menopause" and "the change" but what is it exactly? Aside from the cessation of menstruation, what's really going on?

MENOPAUSE AND ITS FRIEND PERI

Just as menarche (a woman's first period) signals the beginning of her child-bearing years, menopause (the ceasing of menstruation) marks the completion of that time of life. It's part of the natural rhythm of a woman's life. As the process begins, the body starts undergoing a number of changes. There are physical changes in hormonal levels, changes in sleep patterns, appetite, sexual desire, changes in your cycle and more. You may also experience changes in mood, in your desire to do things and even in your relationships. It's a process of becoming who you will be in the next phase of your life.

"Hold on a minute! I'm not that old yet!" Well, you might be.

PERIMENOPAUSE

One of the biggest misconceptions about menopause is that it's a "hard stop" – meaning we go to bed one night, and when we wake up in the morning, voila! We're in menopause. Thankfully mother nature is a little more gentle on us.

The process generally starts several years before the final menstrual cycle. The onset of these early changes is what is known as *perimenopause*. It is your signal that the journey towards menopause has begun.

The onset of perimenopause can vary widely. For some women, the changes occur quickly over a few years. For others, it's a longer journey. Perimenopause can begin as early as the thirties or as late as the fifties. On average, most women begin perimenopause in their mid-.

So what are the signs that perimenopause has arrived? Most women will experience at least some of these symptoms:

- Hot flashes
- Decreased sex drive
- Worsening premenstrual symptoms
- Irregular periods or significant changes in your periods
- Low energy or fatigue
- Brain fog
- Vaginal dryness
- Mood swings
- Poor sleep
- Hair and/or skin changes

Not every woman will experience every one of these changes. Most will experience some of them to varying degrees.

So, why does this happen?

As we age, our physical body ages with us. As we go through our childbearing years, our reproductive organs work hard each month. Via hormonal signals and the wonders of the human body, the body prepares for the possibility of a pregnancy each month. As we age, that capability begins to wane. Our hormone levels, estrogen in particular, begin to decrease. It is this reduction in hormones that serves as the signal that the menopausal process is beginning.

Aside from regulating our reproductive cycles, our hormones also play a part in our other bodily functions. Hair, skin, bone and heart health, our moods, our sleep, our sex drive and more are all affected by our biochemistry. Even our brain function relies on a balance of hormones and neurochemicals to keep us sharp and clear-headed. When hormones dip, brain fog steps in.

Changes like these are usually what send us running to our gynecologist praying for relief. We will talk about this more in later chapters but do know this: there are things you can do and things your physician can offer to help you through the process. Don't be afraid to ask.

One of the issues that often brings perimenopausal women to see me is the major disruption in their period cycle. For years you might have had a period that's shown up as punctual as the six o'clock news. Then, all of a sudden, for some women, their periods decide to play hide-and-seek, showing up when and how they feel like it. That's so frustrating! For other women, their periods become irregular and sometimes very heavy. These are absolutely issues you want to discuss with your women's healthcare specialist especially if your periods are especially heavy or prolonged.

With this drop in estrogen and fertility, you may be tempted to think that your risk of pregnancy has passed. Don't be fooled! I can't tell you how many women in their forties I've seen over the years who thought they were done with raising their family and having to worry about contraception – only to have a surprise pregnancy and having to start all over again! During perimenopause, your ovaries may still be producing viable eggs, and there may be enough estrogen in your body to support a pregnancy. To avoid being surprised, continue to use your birth control or speak to your doctor about what method may be appropriate for you given your set of symptoms and needs.

So, now I've introduced you to perimenopause. She hangs around for a good while, often several years. As time goes on, hormone levels continue to fall, and your ovaries slow their function. You will gradually reach a point where your period stops completely. Congratulations, you've officially reached menopause!

HELLO MENOPAUSE!

Menopause is defined as the ceasing of menstruation and is marked by your final period. How do you know it's your final period? Good question. Menopause is confirmed when you have no period for 12 consecutive months. Your ovaries can be tricky. You may go six or seven months period-free, then, hello my little friend! Still in peri. But rest assured, there will come a time when your period stops.

During this time and later, you may continue to experience some of the same symptoms as in perimenopause. The actual occurrence of menopause isn't like flipping a switch and, "ok, we're done!" It is a gradual process that eases over time.

Once your body has ceased making estrogen, your periods will stop but changes in your body will continue. This is the time in your life when you will need to pay attention to things like bone health, heart health, breast health, diet and exercise (all the things we cover in this book). You'll probably experience some changes in mood, in outlook and in relationships. Moving forward, you will likely make changes that are more in tune with who you are becoming as a fully mature woman.

AND FINALLY, YOU ARE POST-MENOPAUSAL

Once you have officially confirmed menopause, you are now what doctors refer to as post-menopausal. All that means is that your menopause (ceasing of menstruation) is complete and confirmed.

Even though your periods have ceased, you may continue to experience a number of symptoms that you've had during perimenopause and up to menopause. Things like hot flashes, vaginal dryness, night sweats, sleep disturbance and mood swings can continue on for several years. Don't worry, I'll help you deal with those things and more in later chapters.

The period after menopause is the time when you will *really need to take good care of yourself*. Your body has all but ceased making its own estrogen and other reproductive hormones. You may or may not opt for hormone replacement therapy (HRT). Estrogen, in particular, plays a huge role in many of your body's functions and its loss affects how your body reacts.

With the loss of estrogen, women become at greater risk for some specific health issues. Post-menopausal women are at greater risk for things like osteoporosis, bone fractures, high blood pressure and heart issues. Breast health is also a greater concern as we age. While menopause does not cause an increase in breast cancer risk, your risk simply increases with age. The same is true for some other types of health issues, so making sure you're getting your check-ups and screenings becomes even more important now.

Post-menopause is also the time you will be adjusting to life after your child-bearing years. For some women, the loss of their fertility is quite difficult. For other women, this is a time of tremendous personal growth and renewed interest in things set aside earlier in life. You may rekindle old relationships or make new ones, take up horse riding and get your first horse at age 55, take fly fishing lessons from a pro or finally get to take that trip to Provence where you can take immersion French cooking lessons!

You are likely to experience a mix of emotions as the season of your fertility comes to a close. There is no right or wrong way to cope with the menopausal process. You will find your own ways of letting go of what was and embracing the new and exciting life that lies ahead of you!

In the following chapters, we will break down the many facets of menopause and take a closer look at what is happening on a physical level and an emotional/psychological level. We will then take it a step further and show you some real, tried-and-true ways to deal with your symptoms, so you can sail through your transformation process with ease!

A MODERN WOMAN'S GUIDE TO THRIVING THROUGH MIDLIFE

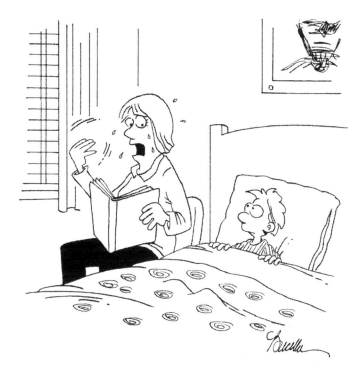

"No, Dear, a 'hot flash' is not a comic book superhero power."

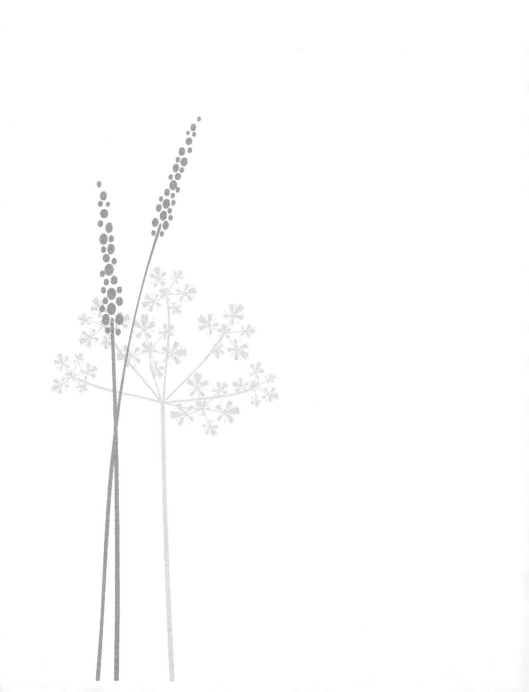

CHAPTER TWO

Myth Busting

"I believe the second half of one's life is meant to be better than the first half. The first half is finding out how you do it. And the second half is enjoying it."

FRANCES LEAR

Of all the changes we go through as adults, none is probably more shrouded in mystery and myth than menopause. Most of us have grown up with some kind of preconceived notion about menopause. Some of that comes from how families dealt with the women in their lives. Some of our ideas may come from our cultural influences. And, then there's the media. Some of what we were/are exposed to is factual, but a lot of it is rooted in history, culture, folklore and a few old wives' tales.

THE MYSTERY OF "THE CHANGE"

For a long time, this time in a woman's life was considered that mysterious time when otherwise rational, reasonable women all of a sudden "lost their minds." The men in their lives would scratch their heads wondering who this crying, moody woman was, and "Where did that sweet, loving lady I married go?"

The kids knew that mommy was sometimes sad. Sometimes she got really upset and would stay in her room. "Who is cooking dinner for us? Is she coming out?"

No one really knew why it happened, but everyone knew that it happened to every woman at some point. It was spoken of only in whispers, if at all. Menopause and women's reproductive issues in general were considered too taboo for conversation.

The medical community didn't quite understand menopause even though it had been recognized at least as far back as the Greek philosopher Aristotle's time. He observed that menopause occurred between 40 and 50 and marked the time when women stopped bearing children.[1] It was generally considered a natural occurrence for women to stop bearing children at midlife.

The ancient Egyptians, on the other hand, saw losing the ability to bear children as a problem to somehow be fixed. Desperate for a solution, it was not unheard of to turn to their pharaoh who was considered a high priest and the representative of their gods on Earth. There is even some reference in the literature to an appeal received by Ramses II requesting divine intervention for a post-menopausal woman. But even a pharaoh was no match for Mother Nature. So misunderstood was the menopausal process that women in ancient times were often considered "bewitched."[2]

Into the Middle Ages, menopause was viewed as a natural occurrence. Much of women's healthcare during that time was primarily provided through monastic care. Remedies for ailments, including menopausal symptoms, were found in herbal supplements, a balanced diet and prayer. Hildegard of Bingen, a 12th century German Benedictine abbess, was one of the first women to write openly about and advocate for women's reproductive health. About menopause, she said,

> "The menses cease in women from the fiftieth year and sometimes in certain ones from the sixtieth when the uterus begins to be enfolded and to contract, so that they are no longer able to conceive."[3]

Interestingly during this time, women who were post-menopausal came to be endowed with more "male" social traits. Having "lost the blood" (menses) previously marking them as impure, irrational or stained, they now gained social status and were more accepted as writers, teachers and leaders.[4]

Moving into the more recent past, the views of women's reproductive issues were at times accepted as natural, sometimes misunderstood and at other times, something to be feared, avoided or managed. As life expectancy increased, more women went through menopause and it became a expected occurrence. That doesn't mean it was considered just an acceptable part of life. On the contrary, post-menopausal women became somewhat invisible and even the target of social scorn and violence.

During the Renaissance, menopausal women were relegated to the periphery of society, no longer considered attractive or desirable. In many cultures, menopausal women were more often linked with witches and witchcraft. In fact, beginning in about 1560 and lasting into the next century, the European witch hunts resulted in the execution of nearly 30,000 women. Historical records suggest that most of these women were of post-menopausal age and lived alone.[5] This was also about the time that the Salem Witch Trials were happening in the New World with similar dynamics. Coincidence? You decide.

Moving into the era of modern medicine, women now living longer were more often seeking medical advice for their ailments including menopause. Physicians of the day were overwhelmingly male and had clear ideas about menopause. Women were starting to look for solutions to what now had a medical name: female climacteric or a fancy name for decreased fertility – menopause.

Not fully understanding the underpinnings of menopause, (male) physicians came up with all manner of ways to treat the woman's waning sex drive (oh yes, women now had an "expert" to seek help from and didn't hesitate), hot flashes and other symptoms. Women endured everything from bloodletting to herbal concoctions known to induce menses, even enemas. (Not sure about the logic there.) This interest in finding the right tonic also gave rise to all kinds of snake oil salesmen eager to sell their magical potion.

Some physicians considered menopause a disease best left untreated.[6] Basically, they had no clue, but, on a positive note, at least they weren't burning anyone at the stake.

So medicine starts to take interest in menopause and along comes the Victoria era and makes menopause a mental illness. During this period, women were often labeled as "hysterical" or "neurotic". Physicians prescribed everything from chemical-laden douches to ovariotomies to clitoridectomies in hopes of removing the offending parts responsible for the woman's "hysteria."[7] After all, what need did we have for our sexual or reproductive organs anymore? We were menopausal and crazy!

There was also a movement to provide women with respite from daily life and give them a place to rest. It became popular for menopausal women to essentially be institutionalized. They were regarded as demented and in need of asylum, but the word of the day was "hysterical." Seclusion in an asylum was thought to help the woman to avoid the dreaded "menopausal dementia."[7]

Pharmaceuticals also emerged around the late-Victorian period. Promising potions including opium and cannabis were often offered to help calm the hysterics.[7] All it really did was create a generation of women who were sedated and hungry. But, the men were sure this meant they had found the cure to these histrionics!

Thankfully, by the time the 20th century arrived, modern medicine started to take women's reproductive health and menopause more seriously. And in 1929, finally, estrogen was discovered by a biochemist named Edward Doisy. (Thank you Mr. Doisy!) This discovery flung open the doors to unlock the mysteries of a woman's reproductive biology and ushered in the possibilities for birth control and symptom relief with hormone replacement therapy.[8] All along, it was the estrogen not hysterics. But, we women knew that already.

WHAT HISTORY TAUGHT US...OR NOT

So now you know some of the history of how menopause and menopausal women were viewed throughout history. Some of it was helpful and accurate, right? A lot of it, though, was not just inaccurate, but downright dangerous. As you were reading the history, did you hear any of the things you were told or believed growing up? Probably.

What we believe about things is often rooted in history, our culture and our experiences. Even though we know so much more about menopause and women's reproductive health today, some of the stereotypes, clichés and old wives tales continue to be woven into the things people think of when they hear menopause. As we continue to learn more and as we bring menopause out of the shadows and call it what it is, those outdated ideas will be replaced…but it takes time. Changing beliefs is slow, but it is happening!

So let's recap. If we were to believe history, what did we learn about menopause and menopausal women? (Get ready to laugh!)

1. Our womb was broken and needed fixing. (Calling all pharaohs)
2. We were witches. Literally.
3. We were stained and impure.
4. Our worth was linked to our child-bearing abilities.
5. We're all hysterical and just a little crazy.
6. Just give us drugs and we'll be fine.
7. But lock us up first.
8. Forget about sex. We're not interested.
9. We don't care how we look anymore.
10. Thank goodness for Edward Doisy.

MAJOR MYTH BUSTING

So with all the myths and assumptions surrounding menopause, let's talk about the facts.

FACT #1: MENOPAUSE IS NOT A MENTAL ILLNESS.

Now, it is true that our moods can be affected by hormonal fluctuations. And, yes, some women may experience depression. However, research has found that the majority of women going through menopause do not seem to have significant issues with depression.[9] What does happen is that mood can be affected by other symptoms that might occur. Hormone fluctuations can cause some mood instability, and yes, we might be more emotional sometimes. We are not crazy. We are not neurotic. We are not hysterical.

FACT #2: MENOPAUSE IS A PROCESS NOT A POINT IN TIME.

The fact is, the changes that set the stage for menopause actually start several years before the point at which periods stop. Known as perimenopause, the years leading up to menopause are the time when we start experiencing changes in our bodies. Onset is generally in the late thirties to early forties. But, it can be a little earlier or a little later depending on the woman's individual health circumstances.

The exception to this fact is menopause following a total hysterectomy. Known as surgical menopause, a total hysterectomy removes the uterus and the ovaries, which immediately ceases the availability of estrogen. For women in this group, menopausal symptoms are more immediate and can be somewhat more intense.[10] You're basically going through menopause in one day as opposed to a few years.

FACT #3: NOT EVERYONE GETS HOT FLASHES.

While the hormonal changes can cause hot flashes, not every woman going through menopause gets them. About 75% of women will experience them but about 25% will not.[11] Within that 75%, the degree of discomfort will vary widely. Sometimes just wearing lighter clothing is sufficient. For others, it is full-on temptation to go lay naked in a snow bank.

FACT #4: MENOPAUSE IS NOT THE END OF LIFE AS YOU KNOW IT. IT'S ACTUALLY A PERFECT OPPORTUNITY TO REINVENT YOURSELF!

Yes, menopause ushers in changes that signal the end of a season of your life. It is also the beginning of the next part of your journey. For many women, the freedom and sense of empowerment that come with this time in their lives is some of the most fulfilling they will experience. Life is what we make it!

FACT #5: YOUR SEX LIFE IS NOT OVER. GET READY FOR THE BEST SEX OF YOUR LIFE.

Many post-menopausal women report that sex during this part of life is some of their most satisfying. Mature women tend to feel more confident and more empowered to be open about their needs and preferences. There are many products to help with the hormonal changes that affect our sexual health (e.g., vaginal dryness), and your healthcare provider can help you make the best choices. More about that in later! And there is no longer the risk of pregnancy. (See Fact #6).

FACT #6: UNTIL MENOPAUSE IS COMPLETE, YOU CAN STILL GET PREGNANT.

We spend a good bit of our child-bearing years trying hard to not get pregnant. Birth control often falls to us to manage. Menopause brings a freedom that you previously didn't have – once your menopause is complete (12 consecutive months of no period), the risk of pregnancy is over. You are free to enjoy sex without fear of a midlife pregnancy.

FACT #7: MENOPAUSE DOES NOT MEAN THAT YOU WILL BE MISERABLE UNTIL IT'S OVER.

Symptoms and how they are experienced is a very subjective thing. Many women experience some symptoms and pass through menopause just fine. Other women really struggle with symptoms and find that they need a lot of medical support. Keeping a positive attitude and surrounding yourself with like-minded people is a very important and powerful way to stay focused on the life you want to build in the years ahead.

FACT #8: MENOPAUSE DOESN'T MEAN YOUR PANTS WON'T FIT ANYMORE.

It is true that as we age, our metabolisms slow a bit and we tend to come up with more excuses for not going to the gym (ahem). However, menopause does not mean that you will gain weight and become a couch potato. As you enter menopause, it is important to be sure that you are getting appropriate nutrition and exercise. This doesn't mean eating leaves and twigs or spending hours in a gym. It means finding the fuel that works optimally for your body and a way of exercising you enjoy. We will be talking about that more in later chapters too.

FACT #9: HORMONE REPLACEMENT THERAPY (HRT) IS NOT ONE-SIZE-FITS-ALL.

Whether or not to go on hormone replacement is a choice to be made with input from your healthcare specialist. You have to weigh the pros and cons. Some women choose HRT and find relief for their symptoms. Some women use it for a brief time. Others opt to avoid it. There is A LOT of information and misinformation out there. It is important to do your homework and have an open dialogue with your specialist. Hormone Replacement Therapy (HRT) is not for everyone…but it's not the devil either.

FACT #10: SEEKING HELP IS A GIFT YOU GIVE YOURSELF.

We are caretakers and nurtures. We tend to brush off our own symptoms and needs while we prioritize those of our loved ones. It's what we do. It is easy to minimize what is happening to you physically and emotionally. The fact is, there ARE things happening. Sometimes really uncomfortable and even embarrassing things. It is not your imagination, and you are not being dramatic. Seeking help is not a sign of weakness but a sign of strength. You cannot be at your best for others if you are not at your best. Seeking help and support is the most loving thing you can do for those you care for and the best gift you can give yourself.

So, we've looked at where we've been, where the beliefs about menopause come from and where we are now. We've debunked some myths and called out the facts. Now it's time to take a closer look at this thing called menopause and what it means in our daily lives.

Now might be a good time to jot down the symptoms or situations related to your own menopause experience that are most important to you. As you read each chapter, make notes. Notice what resonates with you. What questions come up? These are all nuggets of wisdom to help you plan your journey. Ready? Here we go!

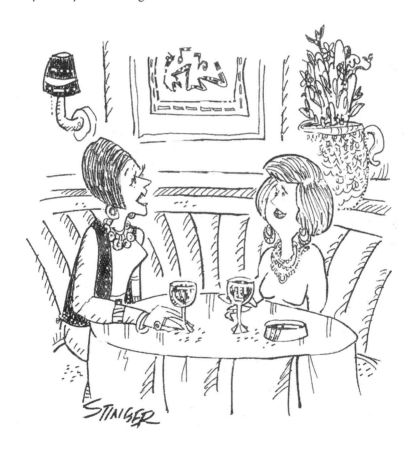

" I'll grow old gracefully when I want to and not any sooner!"

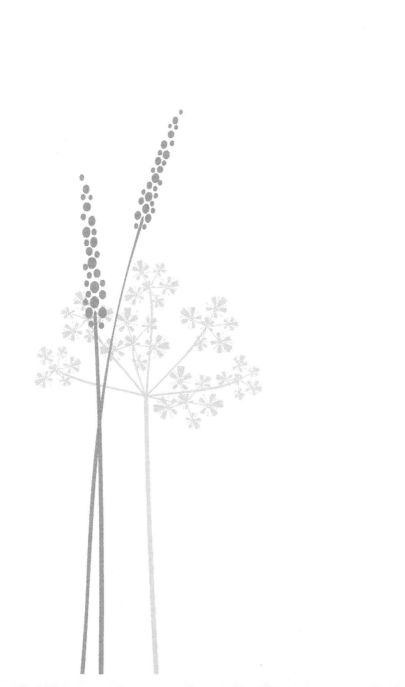

CHAPTER THREE

Am I In Menopause Or ...

"If you obey all the rules, you miss all the fun."
KATHARINE HEPBURN

When we think of menopause, we usually think of hot flashes and our periods stopping. If that's it, then menopause should be a piece of cake, right? Oh, if it were that simple!

In this chapter, we are going to talk a little about the signs that may signal the beginning of your body's preparations for bringing your child-bearing years to a close. Sometimes the signs are as clear as day. Other times, they are merely hints.

As we move forward there is one important thing to keep in mind: women who require hysterectomy with removal of their ovaries (known as an oophorectomy) and experience surgical menopause may experience symptoms more immediately and possibly more intensely that a woman undergoing the process naturally. If you are anticipating a hysterectomy or are recently post-hysterectomy, it is vitally important that you maintain an open dialogue with your women's healthcare provider. You may have specific needs regarding management of symptoms.

WHAT'S HAPPENING TO ME?

You're feeling more tired than usual. All of a sudden your sleep is a mess. Your hair is thinning. Your weight is creeping up despite no changes in your diet. Ugh! Night sweats. What the heck is going on?

If you're a woman in her thirties or early forties, perimenopause might cross your mind. You might even assume that it has arrived. After all, this is the time, right?

Before you assume that your friend perimenopause has arrived, know this. Some of what you might be thinking are early perimenopause symptoms can also be attributed to other ailments including:

- Thyroid problems
- Ovarian failure
- Pregnancy
- Adrenal fatigue
- Sjögren's Syndrome
- High blood pressure
- Medication side effects (e.g., Niacin, Lupron, Tamoxifen, to name a few)

SO, HOW DO YOU KNOW FOR SURE?

I introduced you to perimenopause in an earlier chapter, but because she's so important (and just in case you've forgotten), I'm going to reintroduce her again. Remember she doesn't loudly announce that she's arrived. For most women, perimenopause quietly shows up and starts subtly making changes usually around your late thirties or early forties. It can be a bit earlier. It can be a bit later. The best way to know for sure that you're experiencing perimenopause and not another health condition is to see your doctor.

Your doctor will be able to help you sort out your symptoms and rule out other conditions. You will probably have a physical exam and may have some blood work done.

If your doctor suspects you're in perimenopause, you may undergo some of the following tests:

- pH test – This test involves your doctor taking a swab of your vagina. Normally, the pH of your vagina is about 4.5. This level rises significantly to about 6.0 as you approach menopause.
- FSH level – Follicle-Stimulating Hormone (FSH) is an important hormone that is released by your pituitary gland and is responsible for the growth of ovarian follicles. As we age, FSH levels respond to the diminishing function of the ovaries. While hormone levels fluctuate quite a bit, according to the North American Menopause Society, normal FSH levels in women are in a range from 5 to about 25 mIU/ml. If the level is greater than 30 mIU/ml and still having periods, one is said to be in a perimenopause. If a woman has an FSH level of at least 30 and has not had a period for 12 consecutive months, she is considered to have reached menopause.[12]
- Estrogen – Your doctor may test for levels of estradiol. This is a specific form of estrogen responsible for regulating your menstrual cycle and supporting the function of your reproductive organs. Estrogen also plays a role in many other systems of the body including bone and skin health. Normal estradiol levels are about 25-75 pg/ml. Lower levels of estradiol in conjunction with higher levels of FSH generally indicate that menopause is approaching.[13]
- PicoAMH Elisa Test – This is a relatively new test recently approved by the FDA to measure a hormone called anti-Mullerian hormone (AMH). This hormone plays a critical role in egg production and fertility. Specific to menopause, AMH can help your doctor to predict when you may enter into the menopause process or determine if you have begun menopause. AMH can also help doctors to find reasons for an early onset menopause not due to a surgical menopause.[14]

With all that said, it is important to remember that hormone levels alone won't tell the whole story. As your body prepares for menopause, your hormone levels can fluctuate wildly. It's important to pay attention to the signals your body is sending you and maintain an open dialogue with your doctor.

WHEN THE ANSWER IS YES!

So, you've ruled out other conditions, and you've had your tests. You've met with your healthcare provider and the answer is yes, you're in perimenopause. What now?

First, don't panic! You're not going to suddenly wake up tomorrow as your grandmother. You are not going to lose your mind. Breathe. Acknowledge that your body is changing, and you are moving towards a new season. You're going to be ok.

Next, you want to educate yourself. Reading this book is a great start! Over the coming months and years, you are going to experience many changes in your body. You're going to experience a mix of feelings. Your loved ones might have questions. All normal.

Wait...years? Remember, the process of menopause begins years before menopause officially occurs. The "phasing out" of fertility and childbearing ability is a gradual process. Perimenopause lasts about four to eight years until the process is complete.[15] And, I'm going to keep reminding you that not every woman will experience every symptom or in the same ways. While menopause is biologically driven, it is also highly individualized in how it is experienced.

SO, IF YOU'RE OFFICIALLY IN PERIMENOPAUSE, WHAT CAN YOU EXPECT?

Expect that your body will begin to change a bit. Your routines might change. How you experience things might change. It's all normal and it's all manageable.

Some of the most common symptoms of perimenopause include:

- Hot flashes (the most common symptom)
- Night sweats
- Poor sleep
- Vaginal dryness and atrophy (sounds scary but there is help)
- Irregular periods
- Breast tenderness

- Weight gain
- Loss of bone density
- Loss of skin elasticity and integrity
- Lower sex drive or discomfort during sex
- Changes in lipid profile (higher cholesterol)
- Brain fog

Just looking at that list is scary, right? The good news is that not every woman will experience every symptom. Some of them are just things to be aware of. Others are things to monitor. Still other symptoms are manageable. And some, you may not ever experience.

In the following chapters, we'll take a closer look at these symptoms, and what you can do to manage them successfully. The better prepared and informed you are, the more confidently you can move through the process.

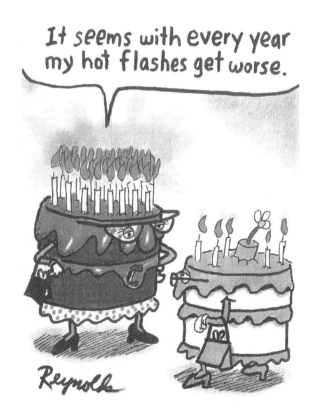

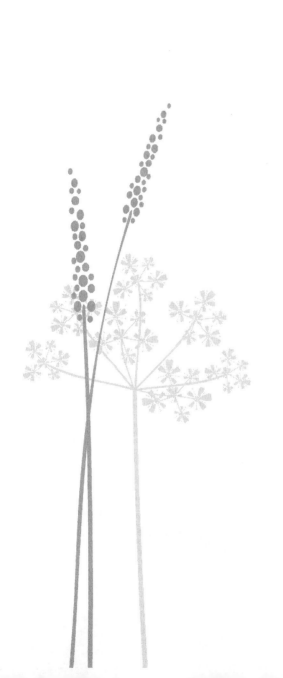

CHAPTER FOUR

But My Body Never Used To Look Like This!

> *"Let me ask you something, in all the years that you have… undressed in front of a gentleman has he ever asked you to leave? Has he ever walked out and left? No? It's because he doesn't care! He's in a room with a naked girl, he just won the lottery. I am so tired of saying no, waking up in the morning and recalling every single thing I ate the day before, counting every calorie I consumed so I know just how much self loathing to take into the shower. I'm going for it. I have no interest in being obese, I'm just through with the guilt. So this is what I'm going to do, I'm going to finish this pizza, and then we are going to go watch the soccer game, and tomorrow we are going to go on a little date and buy ourselves some bigger jeans."*
>
> — Elizabeth Gilbert

Of all the symptoms of menopause, there is probably no symptom more feared and more frustrating than the dreaded weight gain. Or at least the belief that we're going to gain weight. Sure, we're scared of those crazy hot flashes, but we know that light clothing and good A/C can keep them manageable. Weight gain is a whole other story.

Let's be honest. We want to look and feel healthy and fit. We want to feel sexy and desirable. And we don't want our period (or its absence) to get in our way.

As you now know our bodies go through a lot of changes during menopause. Is it inevitable that we must also give up the skinny jeans for stretchy leggings? The answer might surprise you.

FACT VS. FICTION

There is a kind of resignation that many women have that the menopausal weight gain is just something we have to deal with. That there is nothing we can do about it. Even the treatment for it, HRT, makes you fat. Sounds pretty bleak, right? Hold on. Don't trade those skinny jeans in just yet.

It is true that as we age, managing our weight becomes harder. Metabolisms slow down. Appetites change. Ability to exercise changes. Energy levels change.

Enter menopause and we are faced with challenges we may have never had before. All of a sudden, we're dealing with hot flashes, mood disturbances, sleep problems and oh my, our vaginas have lost their minds! Don't even get me started on our bladders and that whole thing.

Menopause also brings along its friends – metabolic problems such as risks for increased body weight especially around the mid-section, insulin resistance and glucose and lipid metabolism disturbances. As a result, the risk of type 2 diabetes, osteoporosis, cardiovascular disease and cancer increase. Thanks, menopause!

But even with all that is happening in our bodies, is weight gain inevitable? Do we just have to settle for stretchy pants? The answer is a resounding no.

MANAGING THE MENOPAUSE MUFFIN TOP

Real talk here: With estrogen in full retreat, your body is going to want to hang on to fat like never before. With that said, you don't have to end up feeling like a busted can of biscuits. You do have to work harder and work smarter to keep things in check. You won't have to starve and the answer does not lie in the latest pill, powder, potion or patch. You will need a plan of attack that you can live with and sustain. Get that in place, and you will still rock those skinny jeans. So, let's make a plan, shall we?

1. Commit – Aging and menopause is what it is. You have to deal with it. And dealing with it means committing. To make lasting changes, you have to make a commitment to yourself and to your plan. You can't put in 50% and expect to get 100% back.
2. Take a hard look – You're going to have to change how you do some things, but before you can change something, you have to know it's a problem. Keep a diary for a week or so. Record everything: what you're eating, when and where you're eating, how you're sleeping, exercise you're doing (or not). Then take a good hard look at what seems to be working for you and what isn't. Those are your change points.
3. Start with your diet – Weight management is about 80% of what you eat and 20% exercise and everything else. Seriously. How you fuel your body and how the food reacts in your body makes a difference. A 200 calorie chicken breast is going to be metabolized differently than a 200 calorie cookie, especially if you are insulin-resistant. While you're deciding on a diet plan, cut out the things you already know don't help your weight loss efforts – packaged/processed foods, cookies, chips, sweets, soda…you get the idea. Just starting there can get you moving in the right direction.
Start looking at eating plans. You're NOT looking for a quick fix. Those are not sustainable and will send you rebounding back to stretchy pants before you can blink. You want a healthy, sustainable plan that fits your lifestyle. Need help? A visit to a nutritionist can be worth its weight in gold especially if you struggle with metabolic issues.
4. Get your move on – Now is the time to start building regular exercise into your days. The American Heart Association and others recommend at least 150 minutes a week of moderate intensity exercise. You don't have to run a marathon or bike until you fall

over. Start with something you're comfortable with and slowly build up. Walking, swimming and biking are all great low impact ways of getting started. The key is to build the habit of doing some kind of intentional movement every day. Your body will thank you.

5. Dial in your sleep – Did you know that one of the strongest predicators of weight gain is sleep or lack thereof? Truth. The hormones that regulate your appetite, leptin and ghrelin, are influenced and set by your sleep time and quality. When your sleep is poor, you are more likely to be hungry and to crave things like carbs and sugar. That craving can be downright overwhelming.

So how can you improve your sleep? It starts with good sleep hygiene – a fancy way of saying preparing for good sleep. Here are some things you can do to improve sleep:

- Create a nighttime routine and stick to it even on the weekends.
- Turn off your electronics about an hour before bed. The blue light messes with your sleep hormones.
- Keep your room dark, cool and comfy.
- Make sure your sheets are a breathable material (skip the satin for now).
- Minimize distractions – use a white noise machine or fan to block out noise.
- Use your bed for sleep and sex only. It is not your office away from the office or a dining table.
- Limit or eliminate caffeine.
- Establish a bedtime and wake time and stick to them even on the weekends.
- Spend a few quiet minutes before bed unwinding – listen to soft music, use a gratitude journal.
- Dim the lights – this signals to your brain it is time for sleep soon and triggers the release of melatonin, the sleep hormone.

If you're really struggling with sleep and you've tried everything, have a conversation with your healthcare provider. Menopause does us no favors in the sleep department. There may be some options to help you get back into a good sleep pattern.

6. Tame your stress – There is nothing like stress to keep you up at night. Every worry of the day will come back to keep you awake. Stress is also linked to overeating. When we're stressed we want comfort foods. And you know, they are usually the soft, creamy, rich things that soothe us. There's also a neurochemical thing that happens in your brain that makes these stress-foods irresistible when we're under pressure.

    It is important to find ways to release and let go of the stressors and worries that drag you down and keep you tense. Find a few minutes each day to just relax into the moment and allow yourself to experience the feeling of peace. Here are some things to try:

    If you only have a few minutes:
    - Disconnect from your electronics for 30 minutes. Use the time for some deep breathing or a short meditation to ground you in the moment.
    - Take a walk.
    - Do some yoga or gentle stretching.

    If you have a little more time:
    - Go see a funny movie. Laughing is a great stress reliever.
    - Get a massage.
    - Go for a swim or just float in the pool.
    - Journal – writing has a tremendous healing and soothing quality. Write about what you're thankful for or what you're letting go today.

7. Consider HRT – The thinking has changed on HRT and now healthcare providers are more willing to help their patients weigh the risks and benefits of HRT. The general rule seems to be the lowest dose for the least amount of time necessary. And women are finally finding some relief from all those bothersome symptoms. They are able to be more active and engaged in their lives. HRT might even help you shed a few pounds if your diet and exercise are on point.

    HRT is not for every woman, but if you're struggling, ask your healthcare provider if it's an option for you.

FIGHT THE GOOD FIGHT BUT LOVE YOURSELF NO MATTER WHAT

At the end of the day, all we can do is all we can do. If you know you're doing your best, then keep at it. When we're trying to change behaviors or keep momentum, consistency is key.

And if you're done with trying to squeeze into your jeans, then embrace your curves! I was recently in Atlanta, Georgia and saw so many incredibly beautiful plus sized women. Their hair, make up and clothing looked incredible – like they had just stepped off the pages of *Vogue*. Their confidence was sky high and so inspiring! My take away from this is that what truly matters is how we feel. Wear clothes that make you feel good about yourself and express who you are – bright colors, fun patterns, soft textures, gorgeous shoes... These wonderful women embraced and flaunted their curves like we all should.

The bottom line is this. Keep it in perspective. Don't let the naysayers tell you this is the way it "has to be." It doesn't – unless you choose it. You can be your absolute best at any age and with some persistence and maybe a little help from your doc, you can be rocking those skinny jeans. And who cares if you can't! Loving ourselves – every part of ourselves – is what really counts!

BUT MY BODY NEVER USED TO LOOK LIKE THIS!

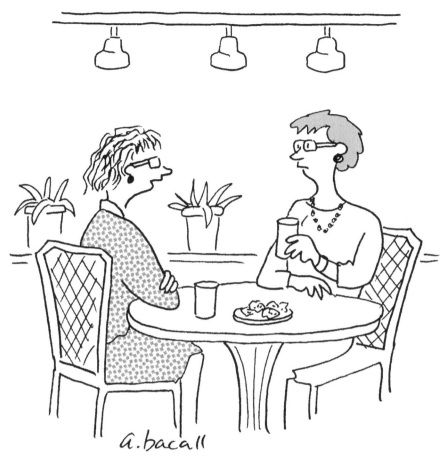

"I started a serious workout program yesterday. So far I missed only one session."

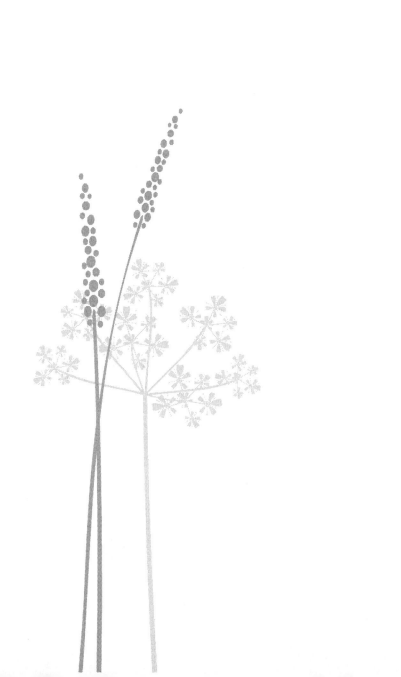

CHAPTER FIVE

Sprouting Silver (Gray Hair, Hair Loss, Changes To Our Scalp)

"I think gray hair is a gift from the moon! When the moon laughs, her eyes produce tears of joy that fall to the earth and onto the tops of people's heads!"

C. JoyBell

You wake up one day and what?! A gray hair...and you look closer. Wait, there's about fifty more! What just happened? I'm not ready for this!

Few changes are more tied to the ideas we have about youth and aging than graying hair. After all, most of us grew up in the age of washing that gray right out of your hair and defying Mother Nature's idea of hair color. We know what waking up to gray hairs means.

Healthy hair is seen as a sign of youth and vibrancy. Our hair color is part of our physical presentation and our overall self-image. It even plays a role in non-verbal communication and how others may perceive us[16] (e.g., redheads have fiery tempers).

Our hair is very much a part of who we are and how we see ourselves. We style it. We color it. We flip it, straighten it, curl it, chop it and decorate it. So when it changes in a way we don't want or expect, it can really throw us for a loop.

Now in all fairness, there are some people who are genetically predisposed to early graying. Others experience premature graying (generally considered before age 30) due to metabolic issues. The reasons for premature graying are not well understood, but it is thought to be the result of autoimmune issues, skin sensitivities or premature aging disorders.[16]

A word of caution here: if you find the changes in your hair are sudden or extreme, by all means, make a visit to your trusted healthcare provider. You want to make sure there is not something underlying happening. If all is ok, then it is probably time to turn your attention to what's happening in your body.

Once we're in our late thirties, we have to look to other reasons for the changes we're seeing. Most often, it's due to our friend perimenopause.

BECAUSE SCIENCE - THE WHY

Graying is a natural part of the aging process. Both men and women experience changes in hair including graying, hair thinning and even loss. But why?

Without getting too "sciency," the life of a single hair begins and ends in the hair follicle. The hair you are sprouting out of your head is actually dead. You have thousands of tiny follicle openings on your scalp, which when the hairs sprout out, makes up your head of hair. Some people have more follicles, some have less.

Hair and how it grows is also affected by your body's chemistry and hormones. Environmental factors (heat, curling irons, dyes, etc.) can also affect its outward appearance. As things begin to change hormonally, hair follicles react and begin to slow down production of hair cells. Some follicles stop producing hair. Hairs become thinner and sparser over time. This is something known as *senescent alopecia*. The follicles also eventually stop producing the melanin that colors your hair. Basically, they get tired.

The same thing happens to men's hair. Men have different hormonal influences and genetic predispositions. They tend to develop something called "male pattern baldness." They tend to lose their hair in a specific pattern.

Women tend to lose their hair in a pattern too. We tend to experience thinning and loss at the crown or sides of our heads or a general thinning of hair. This pattern is sometimes referred to as "female pattern hair loss." It is rare that women will lose all of their hair as more commonly seen with men. When that happens, there may be other issues that need to be addressed such as skin disorders or metabolic factors such as PCOS.[17]

The underlying reasons for hair loss in women are not readily understood, but it seems to be related in part to hormone balance and our friend menopause. Did you know that just like guys, you also have some testosterone surging around in you? Yep, the same kind that makes guys all big and muscly and at risk for hair loss. And it doesn't always play well with estrogen. So as we age, our estrogen is declining and our testosterone can be a bully. Estrogen does provide some protection and has a role in hair growth. It would be easy to blame it on the estrogen since it is the one doing the disappearing act. But, that's only one small piece of the hair loss puzzle. The fact is, our hormones, our genetics, diet, lifestyle and who knows what else all play a part. And as you watch your lovely locks settle into the sink drain, you just want to know what to do.

TAKE CARE OF YOUR HAIR

The most important thing you can do is take care of your hair. What you do and how you do it can have a profound effect on the health of your hair. Remember, your hair follicles are where your live hair cells reside, so it makes sense that what you do for your inside will help to nourish them. What you do for your hair can improve its appearance.

- Maintain a healthy diet. Nourish your hair follicles.
- Hydrate, hydrate, hydrate.
- Exercise and get lots of fresh air.
- Manage your stress levels. Take time to relax.
- Don't smoke.
- Be gentle with your hair. Go easy on flat irons and dryers.
- Use products that moisturize your hair. Leave-in conditioners are your friend.
- Comb or brush your hair gently.

WHAT ABOUT THOSE HAIR GROWTH PRODUCTS?

Watch enough late-night TV and you'll see those ads for growing more hair, thicker hair, fuller hair. When your crowning glory is not so glorious at the moment, the temptation to call that number and whip out that credit card is REAL! Hold on.

This is no criticism to those products, but you have to know what's going on with your hair and what your hair needs are. Just dumping special shampoo on your hair strands may not be what you need. If you're interested in pursuing treatments, a trip to your dermatologist might just be in order.

There are a few treatments for hair thinning that have some support in the research. Treatments targeting hormonal factors have had some success[18] and include:

- Minoxidil
- Spironolactone
- Finasteride
- Estrogen therapy

One of the new kids on the block is something called low level laser therapy (LLLT). This newer technology uses low level laser light delivered to the scalp to stimulate hair growth. It has shown to be effective, especially for people who have not had success with or cannot tolerate standard treatments.[19]

In more extreme cases, hair transplantation remains an option. It has come a long way since the days of visible hair plugs and painful surgeries. Less invasive options include hair enhancements and extensions or restoration.

The bottom line is if you choose a medical or surgical option, do your homework and choose wisely. Of course, you want to look your best, but you don't want to waste your money or feel terrible doing so.

COLOR MY WORLD

Hair color has been around since women were first able to see their reflection. Sometimes we love our natural color. Sometimes we think Mother Nature made a huge mistake. Sometimes we just want to have some fun. Regardless of the reason, coloring hair is readily available and can rapidly become our BFF.

Now, you might choose to embrace your gray. I did (at least initially)! I started turning gray in my early thirties and thought I would embrace my silver threads with pride. But after hearing from many people that it made me look a lot older, I finally decided to find a good colorist and now get my color done every couple of weeks.

If you're not ready to go gray yet, a professional colorist might be the way to go. Gray hair can be resistant to color and colorists know how to get the best result. If you choose to go the DIY route, there are products out there specifically for coloring gray hair. Choose products that are gentle on your hair and always follow the package directions. When in doubt, let the pros handle it.

While you're at it, treat yourself to a professional cut. As your hair changes, the same old cut may not be as flattering anymore. And, as you know, a new cut and color can make a girl feel like a million bucks.

Whether you choose to embrace the grays, go full-on silver or choose a new color, choose the cut and color that makes you feel vibrant and alive. You've still got a lot of living to do!

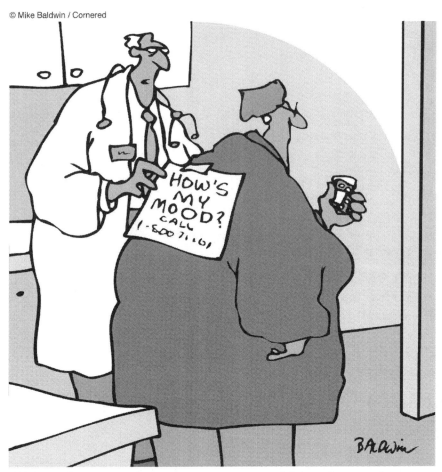

"It's always best to start with a low dose and closely monitor the results."

CHAPTER SIX

Clearing The Brain Fog

"Due to intense brain fog all of my thoughts have been grounded until further notice."

Anonymous

Brain fog. Meno fog. Senior moment. Fuzzy. Yes, we all know the terms. And we all know it when we get it. And it's frustrating.

You walk into the kitchen, open the fridge and… "What am I looking for?" You're trying to remember the name of the song you heard on the radio this morning that had you dancing across the kitchen. That was today, wasn't it?

This foggy forgetfulness is the stuff that menopause jokes and stereotypes are made of. Back in the day, it was kind of just part of the fabric of extended family. We all had that aunt or grandmother who was considered by the family to be silly, goofy or forgetful… even senile. Back in the day, no one knew that brain fog was a real consequence of the aging brain and very much a part of this thing called menopause. Thankfully, today we know so much more and can look back at our female role models with more compassion and understanding.

So, let's call it out and talk about it.

Ah, brain fog. Yes, it's a thing. A very real thing. While it's not a clinical condition, our healthcare providers are well-aware that it exists and know exactly what we mean when we say it. So what is it exactly?

Brain fog is that feeling that something you're trying to remember is "right on the tip of my tongue." You know it and you know you know it. You just can't call it up in that moment. The memory is kind of fuzzy. It's not exactly forgetfulness, but it feels like it. Brain fog can also show up as periods of difficulty concentrating or paying attention to something. These bouts tend to be short-lived. The good news is, it's normal and it happens to all of us.

BRAIN FOG – WHY?

Feeling foggy, fuzzy or not quite as sharp as normal can be due to lots of things.

- Lack of sleep
- Medication side effects
- Dehydration
- Too much stress
- Underlying illness like thyroid disorders, diabetes, depression and others
- Pregnancy
- And yes, menopause

THE MENOPAUSE CONNECTION

As your hormones begin their disappearing act, your body starts to react. You might not think that hormones affect your brain. After all, these are sex hormones, right?

Believe it or not, your hormones, particularly estrogen and even testosterone, have a huge role in how your brain functions.[20] The brain has a ton of what they call estrogen receptors. These receptors collect estrogen that the brain needs.

Estrogen plays a role in:

- Learning and memory
- Neuron growth and survival
- Formation and function of nerve synapses

Testosterone plays a key role in:

- Verbal learning
- Memory

So basically, as these hormones decline, the brain loses some of its ability to function optimally. The good news is that recent research points to estrogen as possibly having the ability to repair certain enzymes in the brain.20 This may explain why some women who opt for hormone replacement report improvement in their brain fog. And, anecdotally, women also report improvement in their brain fog once they become post-menopausal.

Sleep is also a key player in brain fog and even more so during menopause. We already know that sleep gets disrupted during this time. Night sweats and hot flashes and more can keep us up half the night. Not getting enough sleep can leave you feeling groggy, foggy and fuzzy.

WHAT'S A GIRL TO DO?

While we don't know the exact cause of brain fog, we do know that certain things can make it better or worse. If you find that foggy fuzzy feeling is bugging you a little too often, there are things you can do.

First, know that it is a real thing. It is not in your head. You're not losing your memory. Your body is just trying to handle all the changes. Let your family and/or close friends know what's happening. They are probably seeing your struggles and may not understand it. They might have a lot of questions. They might want to help and not know how. That's ok! Talk about it. Ask them for support. And let them help you if you need it. It's not a sign of weakness. We all need a little help sometimes.

Next, take a look at your lifestyle and things you to on a regular basis. You can't change the fact that you're experiencing menopause, but you can control what you do and how you handle it.

Here are some things that can help keep that brain fog in check. Are there some things here you can change?

1. Fish is your friend.
   Omega-3s, those cool fatty acids found in cold water fish like salmon, have been found to improve brain health, nerve function and attention.[21] Not a fish fan? Omega-3s are also found in walnuts and spinach. Bonus: Omega-3s have also been found to help with mood and hot flashes![22]
2. Get good quality sleep.
   We know that sleep is directly related to how we feel and function. Practicing good sleep hygiene can help you to get better zzzz's. Things like turning off electronics earlier in the evening, giving yourself time to wind down, keeping your room cool, quiet and dark and having a regular bedtime routine can help.
3. Get moving.
   Exercise brings oxygen and increased blood flow to our brains. Research has found that regular, moderate exercise has a positive effect on the brain and cognitive function. Bonus: Exercise is also linked to counteracting some effects of the aging process.[23] It's no magic bullet, but why not do what you can? Take a walk, do some yoga, ride your bike. The best exercise for you is the one you'll do.
4. Flex your brain muscle.
   Doing things like solving puzzles helps to keep the brain nimble. Even things like changing your routine, taking a different route to the store and other such changes help too. These kinds of activities call on your brain to work a little harder and keep it sharp.
5. Try meditation.
   Stress can affect your memory. Take time each day to be still and be present in the moment. You don't have to get fancy. Just find a quiet place and simply sit and focus on your breathing. Start simple.

6. Get tricky.
   Sometimes, we need some help to remember things. Make little reminders and use sticky notes. You can also use memory-linking strategies like associating people, places or things with silly images. Or try mnemonics to remember a list of things. Here's a popular example: ROY G BIV can be used to remember the colors of the rainbow. Red, orange, yellow, green, blue, indigo, violet.

If you find your brain fog is particularly annoying, reach out to your healthcare provider. They may be able to offer some other alternatives or want to rule out other conditions that might be contributing. Counseling can help too. Sometimes we just need someone to hear us, not judge us and help us find our way.

The great news is that brain fog is most often just annoying and, take heart, it does get better. At the end of the day, you have to find what works for you.

We all deal with brain fog and we get it! Now let's talk about breasts…

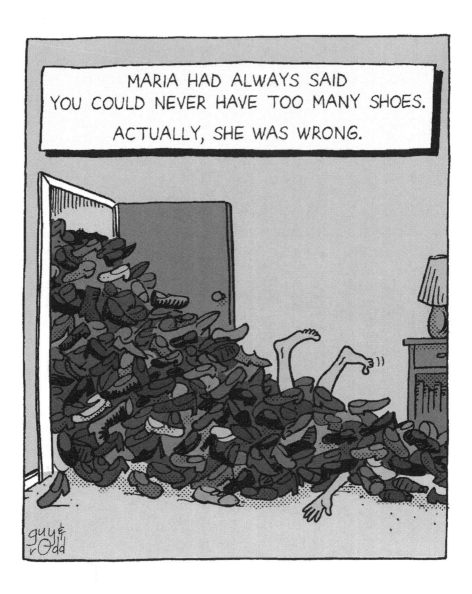

CHAPTER SEVEN

Breast Talk

"I lay on my back one night and looked down at my feet, and I prayed to God. I said, 'God, will you please let me have boobs so big that I can't see my feet when I'm lying down?' God answered my prayers. I had no clue they would fall into my armpits eventually."

Katy Perry

There is possibly no part of our anatomy more visibly associated with being a woman than her breasts. They are the way we feed our newborns. They are the undying fascination of men. Artists have captured them in all their lovely forms for centuries. They are a part of our sexuality. And the very thought of losing them strikes at the very heart of our female souls.

So, let's talk about what menopause means for their well-being.

WHAT'S HAPPENING TO MY BOOBS?

Menopause is an equal opportunity changer. There is literally no part of the body that it doesn't touch in some way. Our boobies are no exception. As our hormone levels begin to wane, breast tissue undergoes changes that can change the way they look and feel. Skin loses its elasticity. "And oh my gosh! Is that a lump?"

Just the thought of it all is hard. But, what's normal? What should you expect?

BREAST PAIN AND TENDERNESS

Just when you thought the ending of your period meant no more sore boobies. You can blame your hormones for this one – estrogen and progesterone are the culprits here.

Now, breast tenderness is nothing new to us girls. It's just part of having our period. But as we start to undergo the changes leading to menopause, it can show up with a vengeance.

Here's what happens: as your period approaches, your breasts tend to fill with fluid and can become tender or even downright sore. The same thing happens when you're in perimenopause. The difference is that with your hormones fluctuating wildly and your period being more unpredictable, breast tenderness can show up at any time. And the pain can be pretty uncomfortable. What's a hormonal boobie to do?

Believe it or not, a good sports bra can be your new best friend. Seriously. There are scientific studies to prove it. Turns out, a well-fitted sports bra was found to significantly reduce mastalgia (the technical term for breast pain) in 85% of the women in the study![24] But there's even more you can do.

The same study also looked at other ways of managing breast pain. The use of relaxation techniques resulted in lower pain levels in about 60% of the participants. The use of NSAID pain relievers were helpful for about 80% of the women. Another effective technique for soothing achy breasts was the use of self-massage using a pain relieving cream.[24]

CHANGES IN APPEARANCE

As you enter into perimenopause, your body is preparing to cease child-bearing functions. One of those critical functions is the production of breast milk. Your breasts' job is to make and hold milk for your baby. When they're in full on ready-for-baby mode, hormones keep the tissue of your breast fatty and dense. When your estrogen begins to fall, the body signals that you no longer need the milk production system and the shutdown begins. The tissues begin to shrink. As that happens, you may notice that your breasts don't appear as full. They may lose their perkiness and sag a bit. Short of a breast lift and push-up bras, what can you do?

The fact is, there is nothing that is going to make your breasts themselves bigger or perkier. However, it may surprise you but one of the best things you can do for your breasts is lift weights. And not just those little pink dumbbells but weight that challenges you.

Why?

Exercise, and in particular weight training, strengthens the muscles in the chest wall. This can help to tone and lift the area making your breasts appear perkier. And wait, there's more! Exercise has been linked to lower rates of breast cancer. Regular exercise reduces the rates of breast cancer in women by as much as 20-30% as compared to women who don't exercise.[25] So grab those weights and pump some iron!

LUMPS AND BUMPS – THE SCARIEST ONE OF ALL

Mention finding a lump in the breast and we all immediately think, "OMG it's cancer!" The tears start to flow and the fear takes over. HOLD ON!

If you're in the throes of perimenopause, it is TOTALLY normal to find some lumps and bumps that you didn't have before. They are NOT likely to be breast cancer. Of course, at any age, when you notice anything that is new or different or just doesn't feel right, you want to see your doctor.

So if the lumps and bumps aren't cancer, what's going on? Cysts are very common in breast tissue. They are simply fluid-filled sacs that may come and go or they might hang around. They can show up at any age. Sometimes we have them and don't even know it.

As we age, our breast tissue gets more fibrous and dense. When this happens, your breasts may feel firmer and rubbery in places. Those spots might be painful at times. Again, not cancerous. Just annoying.

But speaking of breast cancer, let's talk about taking care of "our girls."

KEEPING THE GIRLS HEALTHY AND HAPPY

As you begin the journey into menopause, it is important to maintain your physical health and stay on top of your health screenings. Breast health is no exception.

Before we go any further, it is important to say one thing clearly. Menopause does not cause cancer or increase your risk for cancer. Let's say it again – menopause does not cause cancer.

So why do older women tend to get cancer? The answer seems to be that, excluding genetic predisposition, rates of cancer tend to increase with age. So, the risk of cancer due to aging and the timing of menopause tend to coincide. So, knowing that, let's talk about what we can do to keep our breasts healthy and happy.

TOUCH YOURSELF

Self-breast exams are something that we should all be doing regularly. By getting to know your body and its unique characteristics, you're in a better position to notice any changes as early as possible. According to Johns Hopkins Medicine, about forty percent of diagnosed breast cancers are detected by women who find a lump in their breast.[26] So it's super important to do regular self-exams.

Not familiar with self-exams? Here are the basics:

- Perform the exam the same time each month.
  - If you're premenopausal (still getting your period), you want to do your exam near the end of your period. Your breasts won't be quite as tender, and hormones don't affect the breast tissue as much during this time.
  - If you're post-menopausal, try to do the exam on the same day of each month.
- Do your self-exam in the shower.
- Use circular motions working around your breast. If you're not sure how to do this, the National Breast Cancer Foundation has step by step instructions on their website.[27]
- Perform the exam again the same day lying down.

THE SMOOSH THAT COULD SAVE YOUR LIFE

It's one of the tests that we fear the most. We've heard that it hurts. And honestly, the idea of someone smooshing our boobies between two plates of glass is kind of unnerving! But, the fact is, a mammogram can save your life.

A mammogram is basically an x-ray of the breast. It has the capability to see breast tumors before you can even feel them. It can also show tiny clusters of calcium called microcalcifications. While generally non-cancerous, they can occur in certain patterns that are sometimes the precursors to cancer.[28]

So you might be wondering when you need to start getting mammograms. Recommendations for when vary a bit depending on the organization. The American Cancer Society recommends a screening mammogram every year beginning at age 45. The American College of Obstetricians and Gynecologists (ACOG) recommends offering average-risk patients mammograms beginning at age 40. Still other groups recommend mammograms every two years beginning at age 50 until age 74.[29]

Of course, everyone is different and your health provider can guide you. If you haven't already, now is the time to begin the conversation with your healthcare provider about health screenings you may need including mammograms.

You can't control menopause, but you can do what you can to maintain your health and well-being. A yearly screening is a small inconvenience compared to the peace of mind you'll have knowing your girls are healthy and happy. Now what about your heart…?

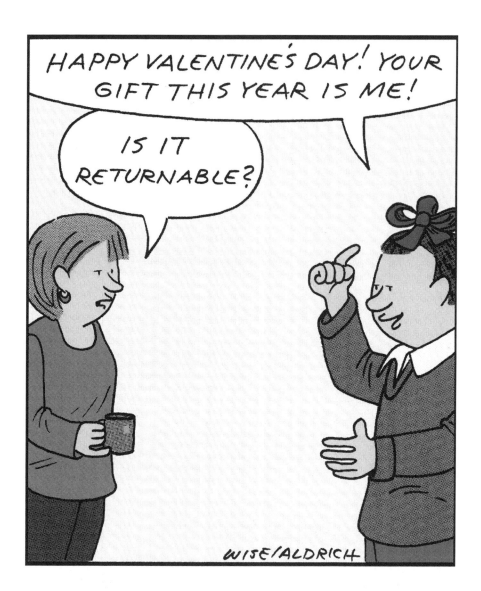

CHAPTER EIGHT

Heart Health

"Your body is a temple, but only if you treat it as one."
ASTRID ALAUDA

When you think of menopause, you probably don't think about your heart. After all, menopause is all about the hormones and fertility, right?

And when we think about cardiovascular disease and heart attacks, we often consider those things "men's issues." Why? Because the majority of cardiovascular events are experienced by men…at least in our early years. But as we age, that playing field levels out.

The statistics are sobering. It is estimated that one in three women has some form of cardiovascular disease. An overall increase in heart attacks among women occurs at about 10 years after menopause. In fact, heart disease is the leading cause of death for women.[30] Surprised? Most of us are when we hear that.

So, if we see that the risk increase after menopause, does that mean menopause causes heart disease? Or is it all coincidence? Or is it something in between?

THE MENOPAUSE CONNECTION

With the rise in cardiovascular issues following menopause, you might be tempted to think that menopause causes heart disease. Easy assumption, right? Well, it isn't quite that simple or that clear.

What we know is menopause is not a disease. It does not cause cardiovascular disease. It is a natural part of the aging process for a woman. What we also know is that heart health issues tend to increase with age. Just like other parts of our body, time takes its toll on your cardiovascular system. So menopause and aging go hand-in-hand. There is a significant increase in cardiovascular disease in women following menopause.[31] Menopause doesn't cause heart problems but it does contribute to changes that can affect heart health. Here's why.

Your hormones, in particular estrogen, have an impact on almost every system in your body. Your cardiovascular system is no exception. Estrogen plays an important role in keeping your blood vessels flexible and healthy so that they can keep your blood moving well. In your younger years, estrogen is one of the things that helps protect and keep your heart healthy, even if our lifestyle is less than stellar. As estrogen levels begin to drop, those protections start to be less available. As that happens, our risk for heart disease escalates. And remember, heart disease is the leading cause of death for women. Not trying to scare you, but we can't change what we don't know needs fixing right?

MENOPAUSE HAPPENS SO WHAT'S THE ANSWER?

Of course, not every single woman will have to deal with heart disease and not every woman is necessarily at the same level of risk. But it is a risk that you need to know is there. And the more you know, the better armed you'll be to make good decisions.

The fact is, there is a lot you can do to reduce the risk of heart disease. You can't eliminate it completely, but you can choose things that support heart health.

When it comes to heart disease and its prevention, the power lies in the numbers. There are specific numbers that are known to indicate an increased or decreased risk of heart issues: total cholesterol, blood pressure, blood sugar, your weight and BMI, even how often you're exercising.

DOING IT BY THE NUMBERS

Do you know your numbers? Do you know what they should be? If you don't, no worries. The American Heart Association has established guidelines for heart disease prevention and risk.[32] Ideally, these are the numbers to strive for:

- Total cholesterol <200 mg/dL
- Blood pressure <120/80 mm Hg
- BMI <25
- Fasting blood sugar <100 mg/dL
- Moderate exercise at least 150 minutes/week
- No smoking

An additional number that has been linked to heart disease is waist circumference. Waist size has been found to be a better predictor of heart disease than weight or BMI. If your waist size is equal to or greater than 35 inches in women and equal to or greater than 40 inches in men, it increases your risk of cardiovascular disease, diabetes, metabolic problems, high blood pressure and abnormal cholesterol.[33]

If you haven't had your numbers checked, now is a great time to do it. You can get a baseline of where you are and know whether there are changes you can make.

WE ARE WHAT WE EAT

You probably remember that saying from childhood. And you know what? It's true. What we eat has been shown to have a direct effect on our bodies and our well-being.

Think about it. What happens when you chomp on a hot pepper? Your tongue burns and you probably break out in a sweat. Coffee peps you up and makes you more alert. Chamomile tea relaxes you. Chocolate makes you feel happy and content. You get the idea. Food does things to us.

What we eat also affects us on a more basic, biochemical level. What we take into our bodies is one of the most powerful influences on our "numbers" and on our overall physical health. Over a century of research tells us that things like saturated fats, refined sugars and processed trans-fat laden foods are linked to obesity and increased cardiovascular disease.

There's also a ton of research that tells us that when we eat in a way that supports health and well-being, we reap the protective benefits.[34,35]

We all kind of know that things like lean meats, fruits, vegetables and such are good for us. But just knowing isn't enough. If that's all it took, we'd all be at our ideal weight and our numbers would be perfect. So why is it so hard?

Our eating habits go back to early childhood. Many of us cook the way our families did. Food is also a part of our culture and our identity. Food is a huge part of the way we socialize. And, food just tastes good. So, when we have to change how we eat, it's more than just calories in, calories out. Our food choices touch the very core of who we are. And change is hard.

What's even harder is knowing what and how to eat. Google "best diet for heart health" and you will literally get 518,000,000 hits. Seriously. How are you supposed to wade through that to find THE diet that works best? Here's some good news: you don't have to.

Researchers have studied dietary habits from every culture and from around the world and seem to keep coming back to a basic foundational diet: lean meats and fish, fruits and vegetables, whole grains and healthy fats like olive oil and avocado. Sound familiar? It goes by a lot of trendy names but it is popularly known as the Mediterranean Diet. There are variations and no single "diet" per se, but the basic premise is to keep saturated fats low, focus on plant based foods, lean protein sources and heart-healthy fats. Study after study has found that this style of diet has a positive and protective effect on the heart. It is particularly helpful in lowering that important LDL number.[36]

To help you get started, the American Heart Association has also issued a set of heart-healthy eating guidelines.[37] Some of their recommendations include:

- Determine how many calories you need to maintain your weight.
- Try to get 150 minutes of moderate of 75 minutes of vigorous physical activity each week.

- Eat a variety of nutritious foods from all the food groups.
- Eat an overall healthy diet that emphasizes:
  - A variety of fruits and vegetables
  - Whole grains
  - Low-fat dairy products
  - Lean meats and fish
  - Nuts and legumes
  - Non-tropical vegetable oils
- Limit saturated fat, trans fat, sodium, red meat, sweets and sugar-sweetened beverages.
- Eat less of the nutrient-poor foods.
- Try to stick to the guidelines when you eat out.

A WORD ABOUT SMOKING – DON'T

There are few habits that are more directly related to heart disease that smoking. According to the National Institutes of Health, smoking causes about 1 in every 5 deaths in the United States alone each year. It is considered the number one preventable cause of death and illness in the United States.[38]

Cigarette smoke contains chemicals that can damage the heart and blood vessels, making it a significant risk factor for heart disease. When smoking is combined with other risk factors such as high cholesterol, obesity or high blood pressure, the risk is even greater. Smoking also puts you at greater risk for peripheral artery disease and stroke.[38]

Now, it's easy to say, "just quit," but the fact is, smoking is one of the hardest habits to break. The good news is, there are lots of great resources, programs, specialized counseling and even effective medications for helping you to break the habit. You want to put a plan in place that addresses both the physical and the psychological effects of nicotine withdrawal. This is a conversation you want to have with your healthcare provider who can help you to determine the safest options for you. The road to smoke-free isn't easy, but your heart is counting on you.

DEAR MENOPAUSE, I DO NOT FEAR YOU!

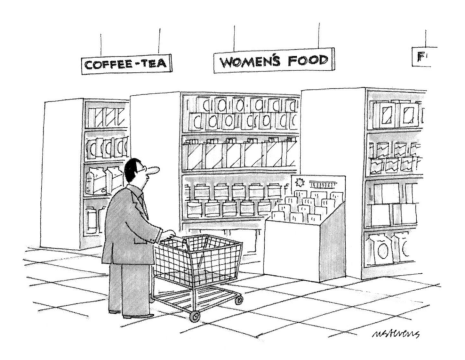

CHAPTER NINE

Taming The Thyroid And Menopause Madness

"A woman must wait for her ovaries to die before she can get her rightful personality back."

FLORENCE KING

Menopause madness…kind of makes you think of that old term "hysterical," doesn't it? Did you know that the root of the word hysterical is from the Greek hysterikos meaning "of the womb"? Yeah, the idea of menopause and madness goes way, way back. From ancient times, they've blamed it on the womb.

Let's be real. Menopause and all its hormonal shenanigans can literally make you feel like you're going crazy. The hot flashes, the night sweats, the moodiness…oh and let's not forget about our period that likes to play cruel jokes on us. It's enough to make an otherwise sane woman lose her mind.

But the fact is, we don't go crazy. And we get though. Now, our bodies… that's another story. Around this time, all kinds of things are happening and some of them are downright confusing. You're cold, you're tired. Your mood is all over the place. What the heck is going on? Is it menopause? Maybe. Maybe not. How do you know?

MEET YOUR THYROID

You've probably heard about your thyroid for a long time. It has a history of being blamed for everything from cold feet to fatigue to weight gain…like we don't experience those things for other reasons. Normally, we don't even give our thyroid a second thought. But when things start changing, it's often the first place we look.

If you've never met your thyroid, you need look no further than your neck. Your thyroid is a small butterfly-shaped gland at the front of your neck just above your collarbone. It secretes various thyroid hormones that regulate metabolism. It's kind of like your body's thermostat.

Sometimes, our thermostat goes on the fritz. When that happens, we start to experience symptoms and sensations that tell us something is amiss.

About 1 in 8 women experience problems with their thyroid. When that occurs, it is usually one of two issues: hyperthyroidism or hypothyroidism.

In hyperthyroidism, the thyroid decides to work overtime. It secretes too much hormone. The most common signs of hyperthyroidism are unplanned weight loss, an enlarged thyroid gland (known as goiter) and bulging eyes. Other symptoms can include hot flashes, palpitations, tachycardia (persistent rapid heartbeat) and poor sleep. Sound familiar? Hold that thought.

Hypothyroidism is just the opposite. The thyroid basically decides it's tired and starts producing less hormone. Signs your thyroid might be slowing down can include fatigue, brain fog, mood swings, weight gain, irregular periods and cold intolerance. Left untreated, hypothyroidism can contribute to high cholesterol, osteoporosis, heart disease and depression. Sounds a lot like perimenopause doesn't it?

So…looking at the symptoms of thyroid dysfunction and comparing them to menopausal symptoms, is it your thyroid or is it menopause? How do you know?

SORTING IT OUT

As you can see, the symptoms of menopause and many of the symptoms of thyroid dysfunction look awfully similar. Both tend to show up around midlife although thyroid issues can occur at any age.

If you're otherwise feeling well, it may be easy to just think your perpetually cold hands are due to thyroid problems. Good deal. Get some meds and you're on your way, right? Hold on there, sista.

On the surface it looks easy to attribute symptoms to one or the other. However, misdiagnosing either one does you no favors. If you have thyroid issues, they need to be addressed. If you are in menopause, you need to know that too and make decisions about how you will address your symptoms.

Although thyroid problems and perimenopause share symptoms, the way the symptoms present can sometimes help you to distinguish between them.

- Always cold – This is the hallmark symptom that everyone associates with hypothyroid symptoms. This type of cold is more than just having cold hands and feet. The kind of cold associated with hypothyroidism is what's often described as a "deep," "down to the core" kind of cold. People with hypothyroidism often have a lower than normal core body temperature and may be bundled up even in the summer. Cold intolerance associated with perimenopause is more of the intermittent cold hands and feet variety. This is caused by stress hormones called catecholamines. Hot flashes can also be followed by a period of chills as the sweat evaporates but it is not due to the thermostat issues associated with thyroid issues.[39]
- Elusive sleep means fatigue – Sleep disturbances are common with both thyroid problems and with perimenopause, but they present very differently. A woman with thyroid issues can't get enough sleep. She may sleep 8, 10 or more hours and still not feel rested. She's tired because she can't get enough sleep. Perimenopausal women can fall asleep ok but will then wake up in the middle of the night for no good reason. Getting back to sleep is hard. She's tired because she's up half the night. Small but important differences.[39]
- Weight gain – Weight gain for no apparent reason can be so frustrating! Weight gain is often seen in perimenopause due to the changes in estrogen and progesterone levels and their impacts on the insulin response in the body. The result is a 10-20 lb average

weight gain for perimenopausal women with fat accumulation most often seen around the waist.[40] (There's that waist circumference thing again!) Thyroid-related weight gain is less specific and may be due to decreased fat-burning efficiency, a decrease in energy and activity or even medication side effects. When weight gain occurs without the telltale core cold, it is more likely due to perimenopause.[39]

- Changes in your cycle – Both perimenopause and thyroid issues can wreak havoc on your menstrual cycle. This one is harder to determine. Both perimenopause and hypothyroidism can cause heavy flow and irregular cycles. What is "regular" is what is regular for you. Hypothyroidism is most often associated with more frequent periods. Hyperthyroidism often results in fewer or no periods.[39,41] If you're perimenopausal, you might be regular but may experience spotting, heavy flow, longer or shorter periods or skip months.[42]

So, that's about as clear as mud, right? If you found yourself saying, "Yeah, but…" a whole lot, you're not alone. Deciphering this dilemma is one that can drive you crazy because one day it looks like perimenopause. The next day it might feel more like a thyroid issue. And still other days, you wonder if it could be both.

SO WHAT'S A COLD, SWEATY AND EXHAUSTED WOMAN TO DO?

Ask the experts. This is one puzzle best left to your healthcare provider. There is no one definitive test for menopause. They can check hormone levels and such, but your history and the clinical presentation of symptoms is generally how your healthcare provider will make that determination. Thyroid dysfunction on the other hand, is something they can actually test for.

Most often, your provider will order a blood test called the TSH (thyroid stimulating hormone) test. The level of TSH in the blood can tell you how well your thyroid is functioning. Ideally, you want your level to be in the high normal range. (The exact number may vary a bit by lab.) If it's normal but you're experiencing symptoms of hypothyroidism, they may order a Free T4 blood test to confirm low thyroid function. If it turns out your thyroid is acting up, your healthcare provider can prescribe medicine to help regulate it and get your thermostat adjusted.

And to answer your question that everyone is thinking: yes, you can have thyroid problems and be in perimenopause at the same time. If this is you, it is even more important that you work closely with your healthcare professional. They can guide you and help you to find the best treatment plan for you.

Who knew that such a tiny, funny looking little gland could create such chaos?

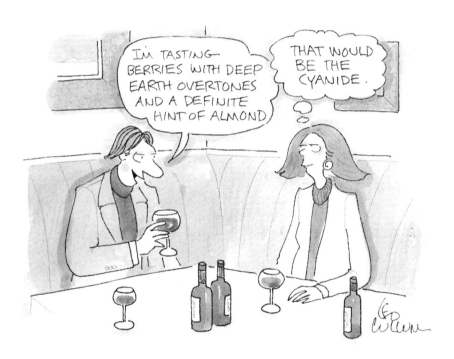

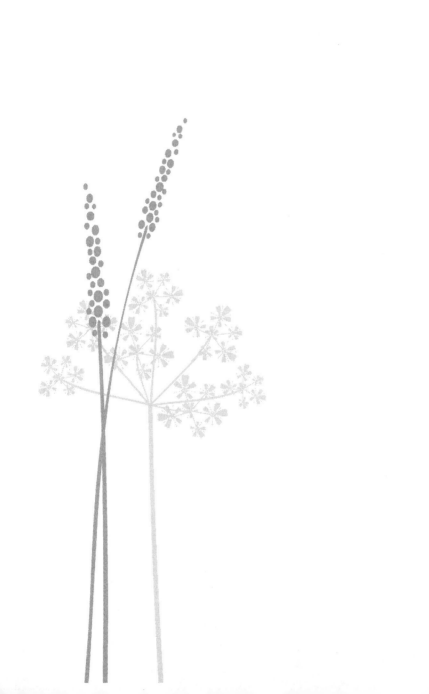

CHAPTER TEN

Getting Your Skin Glow Back

"Skin first. Make-up second. Smile always!"

Unknown

HELLO BEAUTIFUL!

That's what we should be saying to ourselves every day when we look in the mirror. We are beautiful, each in our own way. But as time passes, our appearance starts to change. Our skin starts to lose its glow and dewiness. We start to see little lines and wrinkles.

Ok, we expect that as we age. But, then, something happens. The process seems to kind of speed up. You take good care of your skin but all of a sudden it's different. What's going on?

NATURALLY AGING

Did you know that your skin is the largest and fastest growing organ of your body? It is the protective cover for your muscles, bones and internal organs. It keeps the bad stuff like germs out. Your skin helps keep you warm when it's cold and cool when it's hot. It endures a lot.

From the day you're born, your skin is working hard and time takes its toll. We age as a result of what happens in our body and what happens around us.

- Intrinsic aging – This is the type of aging that results from our cells living and dying. As time goes by, our cells get tired. Our skin loses its elasticity and thins due to a decrease in collagen production. Our hair begins to gray. And our skin starts to get dry.
- Extrinsic aging – This is the type of skin deterioration that is associated with exposure to external factors like sunlight, especially UV rays wind, cigarette smoke, chemicals and various pollutants. Wrinkling, freckling and dark spots reflect the damage caused by this exposure.

So we have normal aging happening and then menopause shows up. And really makes a mess of things.

HERE COMES MENOPAUSE

Menopause actually accelerates the skin's aging processes. Thanks estrogen!

Estrogen plays a huge role in the health and vitality of the skin. Without burying you in the science, estrogen is involved with collagen and elastin production, melanin and skin tone, hair follicle health and growth, the function of sebaceous glands responsible for skin oils and more. As estrogen wanes, these functions slow down or cease. The result is aging skin that has lost its safety net. A double insult. And the skin reacts:

- Loss of collagen (about 30% during the first 5 years of menopause)[43]
- Decrease in the skin's thickness
- Decrease in skin elasticity
- Dry skin
- Fine lines and wrinkles
- Easy bruising due to thinning of skin
- Increase in unwanted facial hair
- Hair loss

GIVE YOUR SKIN SOME TLC

Even though time and menopause can be rough on the skin, there are lots of things you can do to take care of your skin.

- Use a broad-spectrum sunscreen of 30 SPF or higher daily and on all exposed skin
- Use gentle cleansers made for your skin type.
- Wash and exfoliate gently. Scrubbing will irritate your skin.
- Shower in cooler water. Really hot water can be drying.
- Avoid waxing if you find your skin is thinning. Waxing can create tears in thin skin that can be quite painful…and the hair is still there.
- Moisturize, moisturize, moisturize! One with hyaluronic acid or glycerin can be especially helpful.
- Hydrate, hydrate, hydrate. Hydrated skin is healthy skin.
- See a dermatologist regularly to screen for skin cancers and address skin conditions.
- Have any suspicious growths promptly removed. You will have peace of mind that you're doing your best for your health.

A LITTLE HELP FOR US GIRLS

The loss of estrogen can cause our skin to think and become excessively dry, droopy and wrinkled. Skin can become so thin that it tears leaving angry red abrasions that seem to take forever to heal. We can even bruise more easily, and you wake up looking like you were in a cat fight. Other things you likely going to wake up to include dark spots (sometimes called age spots or liver spots), deepening lines and (yikes) hair in the most unwanted places.

The fact is, you can moisturize, use fade creams and pluck or even shave but these are at best temporary fixes. And some of us ladies are not yet ready to look like our grandmothers. What's a young, vibrant midlife lady to do?

See your dermatologist.

You'd be amazed at what is available to us today. Lasers, skin resurfacing and rejuvenation, peels and more. You can even get that stubborn chin hair lasered off forever! There are fillers and non-invasive procedures that can help us to look our best even while the hormonal battle inside us rages on.

Here are some of the most common procedures we can use to rejuvenate our skin:

Botox (botulinum toxin) – Yes, it's a toxin. Botox is injected into fine lines and wrinkles to smooth them out. Injections are fairly are relatively affordable. There are few risks and you're back living life right away. The downside is the effect is temporary – lasting sixty to ninety days typically before you need it again.

Fillers – These materials can plump up areas of your face, reshape the jawline, diminish scars, fill fine, reshape your lips and even fill in those deep lines near the corners of the mouth that only seem to deepen over time. They are absorbed over time and some types of fillers actually act as scaffolding for new collagen growth. They do have to be repeated over time but can last up to two years or more depending on the kind of filler used.

Chemical peels – A scary sounding name but a relatively easy procedure that chemically dissolves the top layer of our skin. Peels can be used to help diminish wrinkles, age spots, skin discolorations and more. An acid solution is applied to the skin, dissolving and removing the thick outer layers. You can get home peel kits but in the case of aging skin, it's best left to the pros.

Microdermabrasion – Basically you're getting your skin micro-blasted with tiny aluminum hydroxide crystals. The result is smoother skin. It's not painful, it's affordable and there's no down time.

Laser therapy – Lasers are one of the most popular procedures for skin enhancement. They can remove moderate to deep lines and wrinkles, improve skin tone, texture and tightness. Lasers are also great for treating certain birthmarks, spider veins and port-wine stains. There are even lasers that can sculpt problem areas where small pockets of fat collect. They can also erase scars and remove that tattoo of your ex that once was so cool. Which type of laser therapy is best for you depends on the needed work.

So now you know, you do not have to settle for skin that makes you look and feel like someone you don't even know. Some of you will prefer au natural, and that is perfectly OK. Others want to stay one step ahead of Mother Nature. Ok too. To each her own – embrace beauty your own way.

CHAPTER ELEVEN

Reclaiming Your Goddess

Vaginas. They're kind of the poster child for menopause. They're where the child-bearing years begin and end. Our vaginas are often what we think of first when we think about menopause and losing our periods. After all, they've been the focus of our attention every single month for the better part of our lives. Is it late? Why is it so heavy? Do I have enough tampons in the bathroom closet?

And sometimes, now that the season of menopause is upon us, we wonder what is going to happen to them when menopause is complete: will my vagina ever be the same?

WHOSE VAGINA IS THIS?

Real talk: menopause is going to change your vagina. Some of the changes will be subtle and barely noticeable. Other changes may make you cringe just a bit. Still others will just be annoying. Everyone will experience changes in their own way.

The good news is, your vagina will still work just fine. Just sans period.

Sadly, when people talk about menopause, they almost never talk about the vagina beyond vaginal dryness. (More about that in a minute.) Even healthcare providers don't always talk about it much beyond that. (Props to those that do! We appreciate you!) So, when you start to see unexpected changes happening, it can freak you out just a little bit. All of a sudden, that vagina is a stranger.

WHAT TO EXPECT

As you would expect, your sex hormones, especially estrogen and progesterone, play a huge role in keeping your vagina healthy and happy. Then, along comes menopause. Hormone levels start their slow descent and time marches on. Over time, you will start to see visible and not-so-visible changes in your genital area and more specifically, your vagina. These changes are not life threatening, but they can be a little unnerving if you're not expecting them. So, here and now, we're going to spill the tea on what to expect in our precious lady parts.

- Changes in pubic hair – This is quite likely the first thing you might notice. Hair grays and thins as we age but diminishing hormones also play a role. You'll notice that your hair down there is graying and becoming sparser. You may also notice underarm and leg hair becoming sparser too. The good news is this change is cosmetic. There is no health issue here. It can just be a bit unnerving if you've sported a dark patch most of your life and now see a gray garden. Bonus: you won't have to lady-scape as often.[44]
- Changes in the vulva, vagina and labia – The vulva and the labia form the outer entrance to the vagina. The vagina is a tube-shaped structure that extends to the entrance to the uterus. As hormones become depleted, these parts can begin to atrophy and droop.[44]
- Vaginal atrophy – This is a big scary name for the thinning and drying of the vaginal walls and surrounding tissues due to the loss of estrogen. The resulting changes can be quite dramatic and distressing. The opening to the vagina, known as the introitus, begins to narrow. The length of the vagina can shrink. The surrounding tissues of the vagina become dry, itchy and easily irritated. Sex can become quite uncomfortable. About 50% of women will experience these symptoms.[45] The changes in the vulva, labia and vagina are collectively known as Vulvovaginal Atrophy or VVA.
- Infection risk – Estrogen helps to keep the vagina's tissues healthy and its natural flora in balance. The loss of protection leaves the vagina and surrounding structures like the urethra at greater risk

for infections. Urinary tract infections, sexually transmitted disease and bacterial vaginosis can more easily intrude and make life really uncomfortable. The good news is, things like vaginal moisturizers, lubricants and vaginal estrogen cremes can help. Sex can really help too to keep tissues supple and less susceptible to abrasions.[44]

- Sexual issues – With the changes happening in the vagina and surrounding tissues, sex can become uncomfortable and for some women, painful. You may also notice a change in your libido. The good news is, there are topical solutions to help with the discomfort. The better news is regular sexual activity can also help to keep tissues pliable and lubricated.[44]
- Genitourinary syndrome of menopause – This term is kind of the new kid on the block. It is a term used to describe several irritating symptoms related to estrogen deficiency that involves changes in the labia, introitus, clitoris, vagina, urethra and bladder. VVA is part of this syndrome.[45]

KEEPING YOUR VAGINA HAPPY

Menopause is clearly rough on your vagina. Literally and figuratively. What's a girl to do?

The most important thing to know is that your sex life is not over. Your vagina is not going to dry up although some days it might feel like a bit parched down there. There are practical solutions that can keep your vaginal tissues healthy, happy and comfortable. And things you can do to keep you sexually vibrant and active.

DEALING WITH VAGINAL ATROPHY (SAGGING)

No one wants to talk about vaginal dryness, itching and irritation not to mention the sagging and drooping that happens in those parts. It can be confusing, embarrassing and frustrating. Talking about it with your doctor can be hard. But talking about it is important. Your doctor can help you to choose products that can alleviate many of the discomforts of vaginal atrophy and dryness including making sex more comfortable.

Treatments for vaginal atrophy and discomfort can include moisturizers, lubricants and transvaginal estrogen. Your healthcare provider can help you decide what's right for your needs.

- Moisturizers – These are applied topically to the vaginal area to provide moisture for the tissues. They are generally over-the-counter and applied a couple times a week.
- Lubricants – As estrogen depletes, we lose the ability to secrete moisture naturally and sometimes we need a little help. Lubricants come to the rescue when you need a lot of moisture like during sex. You can choose water-based, oil-based or silicone lubricants depending on your preference. It can get a little messy but hey, a girl's gotta do what a girl's gotta do, right?
- Local estrogen therapy – This method is used to restore moisture to the vaginal tissues by introducing a low dose of estrogen directly into the vagina. It can be delivered via a ring or cream. These products are obtained from your healthcare provider.

Other things that you can do to minimize discomfort and keep your vagina happy and healthy include:

- Engage in sex regularly (more about that in a minute)
- Avoid douches
- Avoid strong soaps, perfumes and sprays
- Some women find cotton undies helpful, but to each her own

WHEN YOUR VAGINA NEEDS A LITTLE PICK-ME-UP

Your eyes probably just got really big, and you might just have said, "OMG, on my vagina?!" Oh yes, you can now get a little work done on your lady bits. It's a procedure known as vaginal rejuvenation and it is the hottest thing for the well-tended vagina.

According to the American Society of Plastic Surgeons,[46] vaginal rejuvenation actually covers several different procedures. These procedures may be surgical or non-surgical depending on the issue being addressed. You may have heard of some of these procedures:

- Labiaplasty
- Monsplasty
- Vaginoplasty
- Laser treatments to the vaginal area
- Filler injections to specific areas including the G-spot

These procedures may be done for aesthetic reasons (think sagging labia majora) or to address problems such as vaginal laxity, decrease in erotic sensation or urinary incontinence and more. The FDA has issued cautionary statements about some vaginal rejuvenation procedures so you want to choose your surgeon carefully and be sure to discuss all the risks.[47]

SEX AND THE MENOPAUSAL GIRL

When there are changes in your vagina, there are surely changes in sex. Let's be real. The sex we had at 20 is vastly different than the sex we have in our fourties, fifties, sixties and beyond. Oh yes, girlfriends, we are having sex waaaay past our sixties these days. And why not? Losing our period has nothing to do with having sex and some women even find the freedom from worrying about pregnancy downright liberating.

If we let it, the things that happen to our vaginas can put a damper on sex. It does not make us feel all sexy vixen. The good news is with a little patience, a little lubricant and a patient partner, you can be as active sexually as you want to be.

Talking about sex with your partner is important. If you've been together a long time, your partner has undergone some changes too. None of us are who we were. And that's ok. Expect that how you engage in sex may change.

- You may need lubricant.
- You may have to work a little harder for an orgasm.
- Your sex drive may go down…or up.

All normal. Rest assured, if your sex life has historically been good, it is likely to continue to be. Add some spice. Try some new things if you're feeling adventurous.

If you're with someone new, it will be important to share your needs, even the practical ones like using lubricant. It's kind of like the equivalent of the birth control conversation we had with new partners in our early years.

Feeling a little self-conscious or struggling with your new body, pamper yourself a bit. Give yourself permission to be sexy. Buy some sexy lingerie. Listen to music that you find sensual. Allow yourself to connect with your sexual side. Confidence is attractive. Your partner will see you, and everything else won't matter.

RECLAIMING YOUR GODDESS

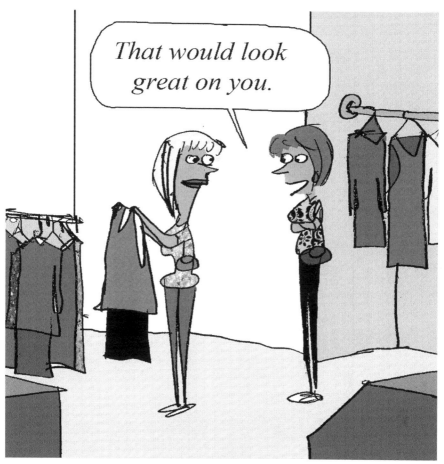

Pam learned the importance of browser support.

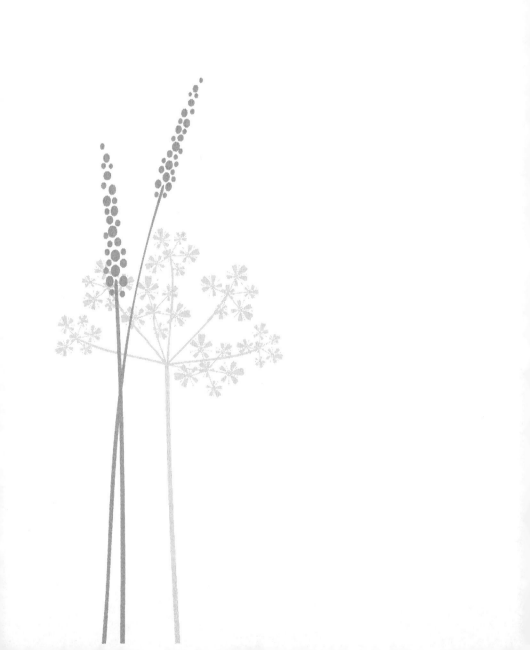

CHAPTER TWELVE

Night Sweats, Hot Flashes And Why We Love AC

"Real women don't have hot flashes they have power surges!"
ANONYMOUS

You're in the grocery store, strolling down the aisles and all of a sudden…

You feel the heat rise and the sweat comes rolling down your face and arms like you've just run a marathon. Is it hot in here?

Aahh, frozen foods aisle to the rescue. And you don't care what you look like standing in front of the frozen peas.

If you've had the experience of a hot flash, you know that there is nothing you wouldn't give for a moment of ice-cold air wafting over you. As we approach menopause, our hormones are all over the place and our thermostat gets all out of whack. Your body is undergoing a million changes and struggling to keep up. Sometimes it gets a little overheated. Welcome to the age of hot flashes.

Of all the changes women experience as they go through menopause, none is probably more talked about, more feared and more joked about than the hot flash. As girls, we all kind of knew that mature ladies (wasn't everyone "older" to us then?) were hot and always fanning themselves. We somehow knew that one day that would be us. Hot flashes are kind of the symbol of or right of passage for women entering into menopause. They can be scary, confusing and uncomfortable. Mostly, they are annoying.

Most women will experience hot flashes and evil twin night sweats at some time during their menopausal journey. For some women, they occur for many years. Other women only experience a few of them. Why that occurs is not really understood. What we do know is that hot flashes are generally seen across cultures, ethnicities and races.

THE ANATOMY OF A HOT FLASH

Hot flashes are that sudden feeling of intense heat or warmth that is accompanied by sweating, flushing and chills. Some women feel it most intensely on their face, neck and chest. Others will feel it over the body. It comes on rapidly and can disappear just as quickly.

Wait, chills? You wouldn't think of chills as part of something called a hot flash. Chills happen as the sweat on your skin begins to evaporate. Depending on how cold the room is, the chills can be pretty intense.

Hot flashes can last anywhere from a few seconds to a few minutes. Occasionally, they can last up to an hour. The average is about one to five minutes. One study found that 87% of women reported daily hot flashes with almost a third experiencing them multiple times a day.[48] And, they stick around for a while. The average length of time for experiencing hot flashes is about four years.[49] Some women experience them for a short time. Others can experience them throughout their menopausal journey and well into post-menopause.

But why do they happen? The truth is, with all that we do know, scientists still don't really understand just why hot flashes happen. We do know that estrogen seems to be a key player. The best guess right now is that as estrogen falls, the part of the brain that helps to regulate body temperature detects too much body heat. It reacts by signaling the body to correct the problem. Hormones are released that increase your heart rate and dilate blood vessels to help cool the body. And do you know how we cool the body? Yup, sweat. It's an efficient system but boy, is it unpleasant!

HELP A SWEATY GIRL OUT!

For sure, hot flashes can show up at the most awkward times! Unfortunately you won't always be somewhere that you can lay down with a fan or stand in front of the frozen peas. You might be at your kid's soccer game. You might be sitting in a meeting at work (Horrors!). You might even be having a hot flash right now. So what's a savvy, sweaty girl to do? You learn to manage them.

SOME THINGS MAKE IT WORSE

One thing we do know is that certain things can make hot flashes and night sweats worse. And they are the usual culprits that seem to make lots of our menopausal symptoms worse:

- Obesity
- Smoking
- Sedentary lifestyle

These are things that you can do something about. If you need help, your healthcare provider can advise you as to what options are best for you. A word about smoking: Smoking is the leading cause of preventable death and one of the hardest addictions to beat. But it is doable! Most people need support to quit and help is out there. The Centers for Disease Control (CDC) has an awesome website chock full of resources and helpful information. Here's the link: **https://www.cdc.gov/tobacco/quit_smoking/how_to_quit/index.htm**

There are also some things that are known to trigger hot flashes. Again, some of these are not really surprising but might be overlooked. Check it out:

- Alcohol
- Spicy foods
- Caffeine
- Stress
- Exposure to heat, as in warm baths or a sauna

Is there anything you would add here? Maybe tea is a trigger for you. Maybe it's chocolate. (Hopefully not!) The point is, learning to pay attention to what precedes your hot flashes can help you find clues to what to avoid or at lease minimize.

LIFESTYLE CHANGES HELP THE CHANGES

You're probably gathering here, managing hot flashes and night sweats is mostly about managing your lifestyle. Everyone is different and you will no doubt find your own things that help and those that don't. Here are some of the lifestyle changes many women find helpful. What works for you? What can you do?

- Be a polar bear – As much as possible, stay cool. Use fans when you need to. Dress in light, loose clothing and breathable fabrics. If you have A/C, keep it at a consistent, comfortable temperature and layer up or down as you need to.
- Chill at night – Night sweats are the thieves of sleep. They can leave you uncomfortable and exhausted. Make sure your sleeping space is cool and comfy. Use a chill pillow or at least a pillow with cooling gel. Make sure your sheets are cool breathable fabric. (Skip the satin. You want comfort.) Keep a lightweight blanket on or nearby for when those chills show up but limit the blankets on the bed.
- Layers are your friend! – Layering your clothing can be a lifesaver. You can go from burning up to freezing in the blink of an eye. And, for you working ladies, you can't strip down to your skivvies in the middle of a meeting, even though the temptation might be strong. Discreetly adding or shedding a layer is the way to go.
- Get moving – It might sound counterintuitive but daily exercise might help moderate hot flashes. We know that regular exercise helps support the body's thermoregulation. It is unclear if exercise directly helps with hot flashes, but it does help to alleviate stress, improve mood and help with weight management. You don't have to run a marathon. Walking, swimming and bike riding can be good choices.

- Just breathe – Relaxation can be your friend during this stressful time in your life. Practice learning to breathe deeply a few minutes each morning and each night. Deep breathing can also help during hot flashes when your heart is racing and you feel like you're going to spontaneously combust. Deep breathing can help calm those anxious feelings.
- Botanicals – There is a lot of anecdotal evidence that things like black cohosh and plant estrogens might have some benefit. More about this later. If you choose this option, be sure to talk with your healthcare provider before adding supplements to avoid any unpleasant interactions or side effects.
- Eat well – Try to maintain a healthy, whole foods based diet. Limit those foods known to heat things up like spicy foods, alcohol, caffeine and such. Pay attention to what makes you feel better and what triggers your hot flashes.
- Stay hydrated – Your body is working hard to regulate itself. Keeping it hydrated helps everything to run a little more efficiently. And, keeping a cool, refreshing bottle of water nearby can be a lifesaver when the sweat beads start to pop.

What if the hot flashes are SO annoying that even all these changes don't help? Your healthcare provider might be able to help. Hormone Replacement Therapy (HRT) can offer many women some relief from hot flashes and other irritating symptoms of menopause such as vaginal dryness and moodiness. If HRT is not for you, there are some other medications that might be just what you need for some short-term relief.

WHEN HOT FLASHES MAKE A CAMEO

Hot flashes don't always happen at the most convenient time. For lots of women, dealing with hot flashes in the workplace can present a unique set of challenges. They can happen anytime and anywhere. You can't call out sick because who knows when these fleeting fickle things will show up? You can't just strip down, and you can't go rogue and take over the office thermostat.

Planning ahead is key and a lot of these things are things you might already be doing.

- Dress in comfortable, office appropriate layers – You may be in multiple places during the day. More than likely you don't have your very own A/C to control. Layers allow you to discreetly adjust your comfort level.
- Enlist an ally – Sometimes having someone who knows what's happening with you can be a lifesaver. If you're in a hot flash situation and need to step away for a minute, let your ally know. He or she (yes, guys really do get it if you tell them) discreetly handle things until you step back in.
- Bring supplies – Smart ladies know that hot flashes often travel in packs. Keep a change of clothes at the office. Keep some body wipes, deodorant and such in case you need to freshen up. There's also a thing called a chill towel that can give you a quick cooling pick-me-up if you need to refresh yourself.
- Use a fan if you can – Fans can really help cool you as well as keep the air circulating. Even a small desktop fan can bring some relief.
- Need to know basis – Depending on what your job is, you may need to let your boss or co-workers what's up, so that if they see you doing certain things, they'll understand or know if they need to lend support. You don't have to tell everyone of course, but you may want to let a few key people know in case you find yourself in a spot. And, it will let them know you're ok. Red-faced and sweating can look like a medical emergency to someone not knowing what's happening.
- Keep a sense of humor – Sometimes despite your best efforts, you're going to have a hot flash right in the middle of the presentation of your life. If that happens, it is NOT the end of the world. Guaranteed the women in the room will empathize and nod knowingly. The men, who may well have wives dealing with it too, will know too. Acknowledge it and continue. They're more interested in your brilliant presentation than a few beads of sweat. And if you can lighten the moment, you'll relax and so will they. Just another day at the office.

As irritating as hot flashes are, the truth is they do eventually go away. In the meantime, do what you can and don't sweat the rest. You're going to be just fine.

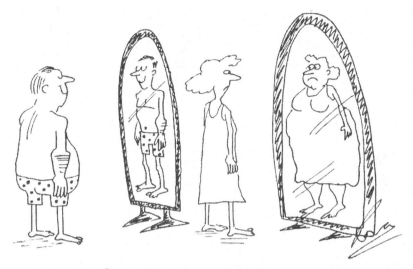

GENDER DIFFERENCES

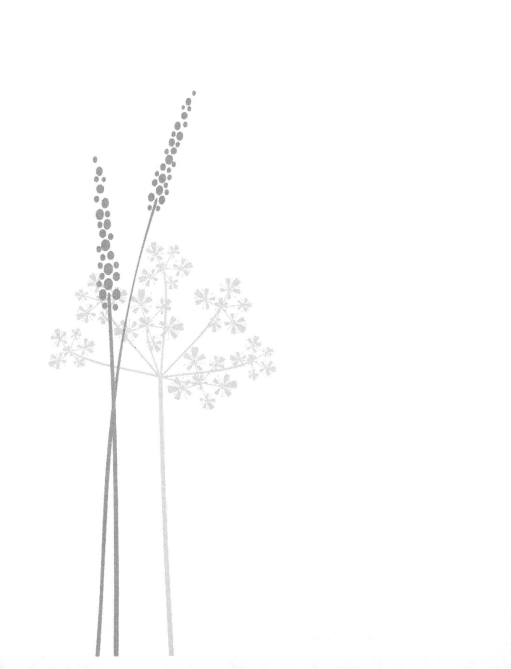

CHAPTER THIRTEEN

Building Strong Bones

*"Here's to strong women. May we know them,
may we be them, may we raise them."*

UNKNOWN

Bone health is something that we, as women, hear a lot about as we get older. Why us? Because like other parts of our body, our bones are not immune to the effects of menopause and the loss of bone density is seen predominantly in women as they age. It happens to men too but not nearly at the rate it does for women.

Our bones provide our bodies with a framework. They help keep us upright and moving. They are super strong. We might be soft and smooth on the outside but we are strong on the inside. The stronger we can stay, the longer we are on our feet.

So what exactly happens to our bones in menopause and what can we do? I'm glad you asked!

WHAT'S ALL THIS ABOUT BONE LOSS?

Our bones are made up of minerals like calcium that help them grow and remain strong. Bone is actually living tissue that is constantly in a state of breaking down and rebuilding. When we are young, we build bone much faster than we lose it. By about age 25 or so, bone-building peaks, and you have the most bone you will ever have. As we age, our bone-building ability slows down. Part of that is due to hormonal changes. Over time, our bone-building struggles to keep up, and we can begin to suffer from some bone density loss if our body draws more calcium that it has stored. Bones can become thinner and weaker.

Sometimes the bone loss can be significant and lead to something called osteopenia. This is the pre-curser to osteoporosis, a disease that causes thinning bones. It can be responsible for weakened and broken bones, limiting or even stealing our mobility.

Some of this loss of bone density is age-related. It just happens. Sometimes there are hereditary factors. For women, our friend estrogen is right in the mix wreaking havoc.

MENOPAUSE AND YOUR BONES

The hormonal gyrations of menopause are known to disrupt your body's bone-building abilities. Estrogen has a bone-protecting quality, so when it starts to fall, our bones become at greater risk. How much risk?

It is estimated that over the course of menopause, women lose about 10% of their bone mass. If there are other risk factors present, it can be as high as 20%![50] Most of that loss occurs in the first few years following confirmed menopause. So, the lesson here is clear. Going into menopause, you want to have your bones as healthy as they can be. Your body will be losing bone faster than it can replace it. For many of us, we have enough reserve. For others, we can't afford to lose a single bit.

KNOW YOUR RISK

So how do you know if you're at risk for bone loss or even osteoporosis? You can't feel or see thinning bones. The best way to determine your bone density is to get something called a bone density test. The most commonly used test is called dual x-ray absorptiometry (DXA) or a DXA scan. The DXA scan is a quick, painless, low-dose x-ray that measures the density or thickness of your bones at the hip and spine. The results are given in something called a T-score that compares your bone density to the average bone density of young healthy adults of the same gender.[51]

A T-score above -1.0 typically represents normal bone mass. Low bone mass (osteopenia) may be identified when your T-score is between -1.0 and -2.5. When your T-score is -2.5 or below, it may be indicative of osteoporosis.[51] If your scores indicate potential bone issues, your healthcare provider will help you to understand what the results mean and what next steps you might want to consider.

KEEPING YOUR STRONG BONES STRONG

So, you've gotten your DXA and your bones are healthy. Especially if you're a woman in or approaching menopause, this is not the time to sit back and wait. This is the time to get busy with a proactive plan to build and preserve as much bone as you possibly can.

Keeping our bones strong requires a combined approach that gives your bones all the things they need to be healthy. It also means being vigilant in protecting your bones from unnecessary injury or wear and tear. So let's talk bone building.

ELIMINATE THE RISKY THINGS

You've seen some of these in previous chapters but they bear repeating. There are a few lifestyle choices we make that can put your bone health at risk:

- Smoking – Smoking affects every system of the body. It is the number one totally preventable cause of death in the U.S.
- Alcohol – Limit your use
- Minimize fall risks – Look at your surroundings. Are there risks like loose rugs, things on the floor? Be mindful of where you step
- Exercise caution – It's great to be active and have fun but be mindful about high risk or high impact activities especially if these are new activities for you

SAVE YOUR BONES!

We can't stop the process of aging but we can minimize the effect it has on bone loss. It is an absolute myth that everyone gets osteoporosis sooner or later. There is a lot you can do to maintain or even build some new bone even before, during or after menopause.

Real talk here: being a warrior for your health takes a plan and some intention. The more you can stay ahead of your body's bone loss, the longer your bones are going to remain strong and healthy. And isn't that the goal?

YOUR DIET

It may seem cliché, but a woman's diet really can have a hugely significant impact on her health. This is especially true during menopause when everything about the body and how it functions is changing.

We know that as we age and enter menopause, our bodies are not as efficient at absorbing and using nutrients as we used to be. For example, bone formation requires a vitamin called vitamin K. Our bodies need vitamin D to help absorb the calcium used in bone building. Women are notoriously deficient in vitamin D. (We will talk more about these when we talk supplements but for now, just know it is a need our bones have.)

Eating a diverse and whole foods based diet gives you nutrients that your body needs to build strong bones. For example, vitamin K can be found in dark, leady greens and in some fermented foods. Vitamin D can be found in oily fish like salmon, eggs, and breakfast cereals fortified with vitamin D. Sources of calcium are things like green, leafy vegetables (but not spinach), nuts, seeds, dried fruit, canned fish with the bones in like sardines and some salmon. Low fat dairy (gotta watch that saturated fat) is also an excellent source.[50]

GET MOVING

Exercise, especially weight-bearing and resistance exercises, are almost universally recommended for building and keeping strong healthy bones.

They have been found to help maintain bone mass and strengthen bones.[52] Movement keeps your bones doing their job and slows the aging process.

Weight-bearing exercises are those exercises that involve using your legs and feet to support your weight. Activities like walking, running and dancing are great ways to strengthen your muscles, joints and bones. It's also a nice cardio boost for your heart.

Resistance exercises are those pumping iron kinds of exercises. These exercises involve using your muscles to push against resistance of some kind. When your muscles pull on your bones, it strengthens your bones. And it might give you some nice biceps.

Right about the time you read "pumping iron," you probably thought, "But I don't want to get big and bulky." Here's the 411 on that: as a woman, you do not have enough testosterone in your body to possible get big and bulky like a man would. You can build muscle, and quite a lot of it, but you cannot and will not end up looking like the Hulk. You won't turn green either.

CURB YOUR STRESS

Mental stress can wreak havoc on so many of our bodies' systems, and bones are no exception. High stress leads to the release of the stress hormone cortisol. Chronic stress means cortisol is coursing through our bodies all the time. And guess what? Mental stress and cortisol have been shown to contribute to bone weakening over time. They might not be the cause of bone loss but every little bit we can do makes a difference.[53]

WHEN LIFESTYLE ISN'T ENOUGH

Sometimes, bone loss or risk of loss is significant and lifestyle changes may not be enough. In those cases, your healthcare provider may recommend a medication to help your body to maintain its bone density. Like any medication, there are risks and benefits. It is an important conversation that you and your provider should have so that you can make a decision that is right for you.

A WORD ABOUT HRT

There is some evidence to suggest that HRT may provide some early protection for your bones. However, the time you really need HRT is in the years after menopause. For a woman with a certain profile, HRT might be a consideration. HRT may be recommended for postmenopausal women who have:[54]

- An early menopause (especially before age 40)
- Low bone mass and menopausal symptoms
- Risk factors for osteoporosis, such as a petite, thin frame; family history or a medical problem associated with osteoporosis

Use of HRT isn't without risks, however.[54] Studies have shown that some types of HRT may increase your risk of developing:

- Breast cancer
- Gallbladder disease
- Blood clots
- High blood pressure (in some women)

Our bones keep us upright and keep us moving. Take good care of your bones, and they will take good care of you.

CHAPTER FOURTEEN

Hormone Therapy Demystified And Why It's Not Right For Everyone

"Women speak in estrogen, and men listen in testosterone."

RICHARD ROEPER

Hormone Replacement Therapy or HRT is one of those topics that always seems to come up whenever women of a certain age are gathered. There's always someone who has had stellar results with it. There's always someone who had awful results. Still, others have all kinds of ideas and notions. Some based in fact. Some not so much.

Over the years, HRT has been lauded as the answer to many a menopausal woman's prayers. At times, it has been demonized as the devil. It's been recommended for all kinds of menopausal and reproductive issues with varying degrees of success.

HRT has come to us in many forms over the years – pills, patches and creams – each with their own unique profile. Yet, we lump it all into the pile that is HRT. So, if it has evolved and it comes in different forms and different combinations, how do we know what works, what doesn't, what helps menopause symptoms and what doesn't? And the even bigger question that we all have, "Is it safe?"

So, we are going to take a deeper dive and look at HRT, what it is and what it's not.

WHAT IS HRT?

Hormone Replacement Therapy or HRT is exactly what it sounds like. HRT is the replacement of the body's naturally occurring female sex hormones, estrogen and progesterone. HRT may consist of estrogen alone or in combination with progesterone. Estrogen and progesterone are also sometimes combined with testosterone. The hormones may be delivered in pill form, in a transdermal patch, vaginal ring, in a cream or gel base and even in a nasal spray.

HRT is most often used to treat menopausal symptoms before age 50 or so. What type of HRT and how long you'll take it is something that you and your healthcare provider will determine. Every woman is different, and HRT is definitely not one size fits all.

HOW IS HRT USED?

The general rule for using HRT is the lowest effective dose for the least amount of time necessary. Basically, HRT can be used to help you get through the roughest parts of menopause, but in most cases, it is not to be used indefinitely.

The American College of Obstetricians and Gynecologists (ACOG), the Endocrine Society and the North American Menopause Society (NAMS) have established guidelines for the use of HRT.

- In women under 60 who are less than 10 years post menopause and have had a hysterectomy, experience hot flashes and have **no contraindications** to HRT or excessive cardiovascular or breast cancer risk, use of estrogen-only therapy is recommended.[55,56]
- In women under 60 who are less than 10 years post menopause and still have an intact uterus, experience irritating hot flashes and have no contraindications to HRT or excessive cardiovascular or breast cancer risk, estrogen with the addition of a progestin is

recommended to prevent endometrial hyperplasia and potential endometrial cancer use.[55,56]
- For women aged older than 60 years or who are more than 10 years post menopause, non-hormonal options are recommended.[55]
- Women with an elevated risk of cardiovascular disease non-hormonal therapies should consider non-hormonal options.[55]
- For women with moderate risk for cardiovascular disease, transdermal estrogen with or without progestin is preferred over oral therapy. Transdermal delivery has less effect on blood pressure, lipids, and carbohydrate metabolism.[57]
- For women with an elevated risk for breast cancer, non-hormonal options are recommended.[56]
- For women who experience early menopause (before age 45 or due to hysterectomy), HRT can be used before age 50 with no increased risk of breast cancer.[57]

Now, even with all those guidelines, what is right for you might not be right for another woman even if her symptoms are similar. In addition to a medical profile, you also have to look at lifestyle, heredity factors, other medications and conditions and even fears about using HRT. This is why before deciding on HRT, it is so important to have conversations with your healthcare provider and ask lots of questions.

THE DOWNSIDE TO HRT

HRT is, in fact, a medical intervention. You are introducing medically manufactured and medically prescribed substances into your body. There are bound to be side effects. They can range from irritating to downright dangerous. Not everyone will experience every side effect. But you need to know that they exist so that you can make an informed decision. As the old saying goes, forewarned is forearmed.

Major side effects associated with HRT include:

- Increased risk of cardiovascular disease
- Increased risk of breast cancer

- Increased risk of endometrial or ovarian cancer in women with an intact uterus and ovaries
- Stroke
- Blood clots
- Increased risk of endometrial hyperplasia and cancer in women with a uterus who use estrogen only
- Some risk of developing breast cancer when a woman is on estrogen for 5 years[56]

Patients who are over age 60 or who are more than 10 years from the start of menopause seem to be at greatest risk for these negative effects. You and your doctor have to weigh the risks and benefits. But before you make a decision, you always want to be informed and make the decision that is right for your situation.

IS HRT FOR ME?

Whether or not HRT is for you or not is a two-sided decision. First, there is the medical picture. Is your situation appropriate for HRT, or are you at a higher risk for side effects?

WHO SHOULD NOT TAKE HRT?

Although there are no absolutes, experts generally agree[55,56,57] that HRT should be avoided in women with:

- Unexplained vaginal bleeding
- History of stroke or transient ischemic attack
- Heart attack
- Pulmonary embolism or VTE
- Breast or endometrial cancer
- Active liver disease
- Known protein C, protein S or clotting disorders
- Known or suspected pregnancy

- Caution should be exercised in patients with diabetes, gallbladder disease, hypertriglyceridemia (>400 mg/day), hypoparathyroidism, high risk for breast cancer, high risk for heart disease or migraine with aura.

The other thing to consider is how you feel about HRT. Are you comfortable with the risk vs. benefit? Will you be compliant with the treatment plan? Does HRT conflict with your lifestyle philosophy or way of living? You have to be confident in your decisions about your body.

Know this…If HRT is not for you, that's ok too. There are non-hormonal, natural alternatives that you can explore, and we are going to talk about them next.

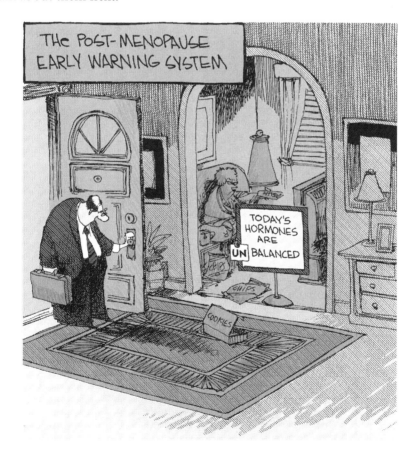

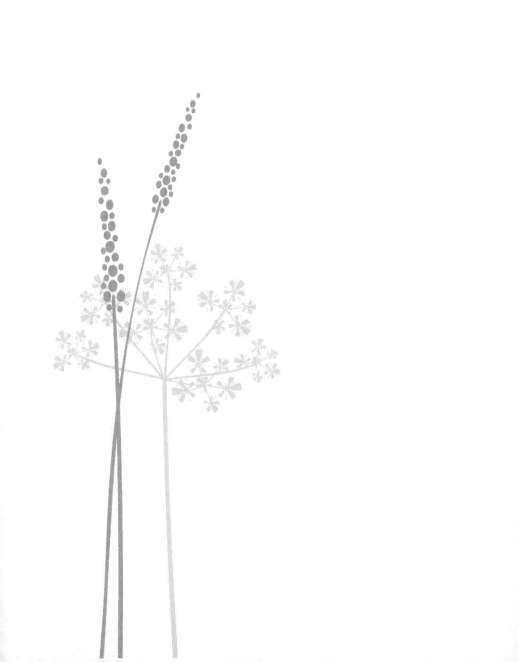

CHAPTER FIFTEEN

When East Meets West – Understanding The Best Natural Therapies To Help You

"The art of healing comes from nature, not from the physician. Therefore the physician must start from nature, with an open mind."
Paracelsus

Alternative therapies, alternative medicine, Eastern practices…

Whatever tag you give it, medicine and alternative practices have been around for thousands of years. They're nothing new. What is new is the interest that people have for alternatives to traditional Western medicine. More and more, people are seeking non-medical ways of treating their health issues. And what they're finding in a lot of cases is relief.

What was once dismissed as a bunch of hooey is now being touted as one more powerful tool in treating the whole person. What we're learning is what many people have known anecdotally for centuries. There is a healing force in nature that can't be easily explained by Western medicine. Sometimes the best medicine isn't medicine at all but rather an understanding of the body as a whole. Eastern tradition is meeting Western medicine and together, they are becoming a powerful force in healthcare.

So what are we talking about here? Needles between the eyes? Drinking mixtures of secret herbs and spices? Well, sort of but not really. What we're talking about are practices that are steeped in Eastern traditions, folk medicine and such as well as things like psychotherapy and expressive arts. You don't have to get needles but guess what? Acupuncture is on the list.

ALTERNATIVE THERAPIES MEET MENOPAUSE

Not unexpectedly, there is a significant concern about the use of HRT in treating the symptoms of menopause. Some of that concern is founded. Some of it may be fear. It might simply be a desire to embrace the healing power of nature. Whatever the reason, women are turning to alternative or complimentary therapies to find relief. In fact, a recent survey found that 95% of the women surveyed said they would try an alternative therapy before trying HRT, citing concerns about HRT risks and a desire to try a natural alternative.[58]

Researchers have taken notice, and they are now taking a hard look at what, besides HRT, works for menopause symptoms. Even the UK's National Institute for Health and Care Excellence (NICE) is using evidence-based criteria to compare popular alternative therapies with HRT.[59] And what they're finding might surprise you.

So, without further ado, let's see what all this alternative stuff is about.

ACUPUNCTURE

Acupuncture is a holistic therapy rooted in traditional Chinese medicine. Fine needles are used to stimulate certain points in the body to balance the flow of energy and promote healing. It has tons of anecdotal evidence of effectiveness from people who use it. It's been around for thousands of years and used for a myriad of ailments. When it comes to menopause, it might just be something to take a look at. Recent research found that acupuncture resulted in rapid and clinically significant reduction in hot flashes during the six-week intervention. No severe adverse effects were reported.[60] WOW! Other studies have found similar results. So, if you're not needle phobic, acupuncture might be one to consider. Wondering how to find a licensed acupuncturist? A good place to start is the National Certification Commission for Acupuncture and Oriental Medicine (NCCAOM) https://directory.nccaom.org/home/index.

COGNITIVE BEHAVIORAL THERAPY (CBT)

CBT is a specific type of psychotherapy that helps people learn to modify irritating emotions, behaviors, and thoughts and to develop personal coping strategies. When used to help women deal with menopause symptoms like hot flashes and insomnia, CBT seems to be a winner. Studies have found that a program of CBT can help reduce the intensity of hot flashes and help women better manage them when they happen. Additional benefits of CBT include improved mood, better sleep and improved memory and concentration. What makes this even more tempting is that the benefits seem to persist over time![61] One super interesting study even combined therapy with traditional Chinese medicine. Now that's East meets West! CBT is a popular therapeutic approach so finding a CBT therapist is pretty easy. If you like to talk about your menopause, CBT might be an excellent fit for you.

HYPNOTHERAPY

Hypnotherapy, sometimes referred to trance work, has been around for thousands of years. History is full of examples of its use in various cultures, from the "healing passes" of the Hindu Vedas, to the "magical texts" of ancient Egypt. Hypnotic practices were then used for magical or religious purposes, but it was their way of curing humanity's ills of the day.[68]

Today, hypnosis is used for all sorts of conditions and has even proven effective with reducing menopausal symptoms. Hypnotherapy has been found to reduce the frequency of hot flashes in menopausal women. Study participants also said that hot flashes didn't interfere with their lives as much and they slept better.[69] Reduces hot flashes and improves sleep? Sign me up!

STRESS MANAGEMENT

High levels of stress are correlated with as many as 50-80% of all diseases. Stress contributes to suppression of the immune system; susceptibility to illness, particularly to immune-related disorders and cancer; high blood pressure; increased blood levels of cholesterol and depletion of vitamins and minerals. So it would make sense that reducing stress could help to improve menopausal symptoms. And research agrees.

A number of studies have found that use of various relaxation techniques result a reduction of hot flashes. One study found that relaxation and deep breathing helped to reduce the severity of hot flashes by as much as 50%.[62] These relaxation techniques also have been shown to help reduce the severity of other symptoms. Relaxation techniques are simple, easy to learn and you can do them anywhere. Sometimes all you need is a few minutes and a few deep breaths.

TRADITIONAL EASTERN HERBAL MEDICINE

Herbal remedies have long been a cornerstone to treating women's menopausal symptoms. Before there was HRT, there was herbal medicine. Different practices emerged in different parts of the world using herbs that were available to them and based on the local traditions and influences. Eastern herbal medicine originates from traditional Asian or Indian practices and are rooted in traditional Chinese, Japanese or Ayurvedic approaches.

Herbal remedies are interesting because they are based on the unique needs of the woman being tended to. Although two women may be seeking relief from hot flashes, their herbal prescriptions will contain a blend of herbs formulated for her own unique biochemical needs.

Interestingly, there is some overlap between East and West here. Both camps agree that compounds like phytoestrogens can reduce menopausal symptoms. In Chinese medicine, food is considered medicine and prescriptions might include phytoestrogen-rich foods like tofu. Ginseng and Dang Kui are herbs that are known to relieve symptoms of menopause.[63]

So we know what history and tradition say. Thousands of years can't be wrong, right? But what does science say? Well, it's mixed. Some studies are inconclusive.[64] Other studies support this treatment alternative.[65] It doesn't mean these traditional medicine practices don't work. On the contrary, there's thousands of years of practice and anecdotal evidence behind them. However, when studied using Western scientific models, there isn't clear evidence that they do help. It may very well be that whether this method helps or not is a highly individualized response to a highly individualized prescription of herbs. Don't write this one off. If you find this traditional herbal medicine interesting, you may want to seek out a practitioner and try it.

OTHER HERBAL REMEDIES

There are other various herbal remedies that have been used for thousands of years by women around the world. Again, before there was HRT, women had to fend for themselves and find relief where they could. They relied heavily on the folk medicine of their culture. Many of these herbal supplements and their uses were passed down from mother to daughter and from woman to woman. Some have stood the test of time and are still used today. There are literally hundreds of herbs and concoctions that folk medicine practitioners have used. Let's take a look at some of the more popular ones.

Black Cohosh – This herb is actually a member of the buttercup family and has been used by Native American and Chinese herbal practices. Black cohosh has quite the reputation for being a hot flash smasher. According to the National Center for Complementary and Integrative Health, studies of black cohosh's effectiveness for treating menopausal symptoms have been mixed on whether it's effective but many women swear by it.[66] It is widely available in drug stores, so it's easy to try it for yourself. You may be one of the women that has a positive response.

St. John's Wort – This herbal powerhouse has been used in herbal medicine as far back as ancient Greece. Historically touted as a natural anti-depressant, St. John's Wort has also been shown to be effective in reducing hot flashes as well as the depression that can sometimes accompany the transition to menopause.[67] This herb is known to have some negative interactions with some drugs so if you're going to try it, be sure you are talking with your healthcare provider. You don't want any surprises.

There are many, many other herbs that have anecdotal evidence but are just not backed up by scientific evidence. Evening primrose oil, ginseng, red clover and others are herbs that may be helpful to some people in some blends. The bottom line with herbal alternatives seems to be this: be cautious and be careful. Do your homework and talk openly with your healthcare provider. Information is your friend. Yes, you want relief, but you also want get relief safely. If you have all the information and the green light from your healthcare provider, you may want to try an herbal approach. But do so safely by knowing the risks.

CHAPTER SIXTEEN

Meditation, Yoga, Pilates And Other Ways To Transform Body And Spirit

"When you begin to meditate on a regular basis, you will start to notice that thoughts and feelings that may have been building up inside of you are gently released and you reach the quiet place that was always there, waiting for you – the place of pure awareness. It is there that you will experience peace, healing, and true rejuvenation."

Deepak Chopra

Going through the process of menopause is not just a challenge in managing the symptoms. It's a challenge of redefining and reconnecting with who we are, finding peace with where we are in life and what comes next. This journey can be overwhelming. Sometimes it can seem like we are just one big hot flash. When that happens, our head and our heart, our mind and our body are distressed. And it's exhausting. That's about to change. Right here, right now.

THE MIND-BODY CONNECTION

Much has been written about the mind-body connection and how important it is to our well-being. But do you know what it really means? If you had to describe it in 25 words or less, could you? Don't worry, most people can't.

The mind-body connection is the dynamic between mental health and physical health. It is the connection through which emotional, psychological and behavioral factors (mind) can directly affect physical health (body) outcomes. What you think, feel and believe about yourself and the world around you can have a profound effect on your health and well-being. How does this happen? Neurotransmitters and neural pathways. Those are fancy terms for how your mind and your body talk to each other.

Your mental state can have a positive or negative effect on our physical/biological functions. So, when you're feeling frustrated or angry about something, say yet another embarrassing hot flash, your "mind" is communicating to your "body" that it's upset and feeling all kinds of negativity via the release of neurotransmitters that travel along these pathways. Your body may respond with an increase in tension or anxiety or even physical pain like a headache.

So why is this so important to menopause? Because the way you approach menopause, your feelings and thoughts about it, can affect your body, your symptoms or even compromise your health in other ways. Research tells us that mindset plays a huge role in managing symptoms of menopause.[70] We are also learning that mind-body practices can help protect and improve sleep (always an issue with menopause) as well as mitigate specific symptoms of menopause like hot flashes, stress and depression.[71] And bonus, these kinds of activities are just soothing. When you find the one that speaks to you, you're going to want to do it all the time.

So now you know what the mind-body connection is all about. Now let's talk about how to build that connection using practices that promote mind-body connection and are beneficial for women dealing with menopause. Some of these are very popular and you might already be doing some of them. If so, keep doing what works. If you're new to these, don't be intimidated. These methods are all super easy to do, adaptable to your abilities and most require nothing more than space to spread out. Ready?

YOGA

No surprise with this one. Yoga, in all its forms, has been around for literally thousands of years and has its roots in ancient Indian philosophy. Yoga combines various physical postures (poses) and movement, breathing techniques and meditation to calm the mind and increase awareness of the moment. It can be intense or gentle, fast or slow depending on the type of yoga you choose.

Yoga has been found to reduce the intensity of hot flashes and night sweats as well as help women to feel less bothered by them. Yoga has a positive effect on sleep, stress levels and lowered levels of anxiety and depression.[71]

MINDFULNESS MEDITATION

Mindfulness meditation is a type of meditation that involves completely focusing on the present moment. The here-and-now. It is a simple practice that can be done almost anywhere. All you need is a few quiet moments. Here's a quick mindfulness practice that I've found particularly helpful when I'm feeling overwhelmed:

> *Stop what you're doing, sit in a comfy chair and close your eyes. Place your hands gently in your lap. Now take a deep breath in, hold and let it go. Do this several more times. As you're breathing deeply, focus on the sound of your breathing. If something distracts you, gently brush it aside in your mind and return your attention to your breathing. Now, just breathe naturally. Again, focus on the sounds of your breathing – in and out. One more deep breath, and now slowly open your eyes.*

Congratulations, you just did a simple mindfulness meditation!

There are lots of meditation styles and there is no "one way." Do what works for you.

It's hard to imagine that something so simple can be so powerful but it is. Mindfulness meditation has been shown to significantly improve the psychological aspects of coping with menopausal symptoms. While the results for reducing hot flashes are mixed,[72] mindfulness meditation has shown to reduce the level of "bother" that women feel with hot flashes. They just weren't that bothered by them when they happened. Mood, anxiety and sleep improved too.[73]

PILATES

When we think of therapies for menopause, Pilates might not immediately come to mind. Pilates is often associated with muscle strengthening and flexibility. But given the physical impact menopause can have on our bones and tissues, Pilates makes perfect sense. Pilates can improve core strength, muscle strength and balance all with little joint impact. But does it specifically help with symptoms of menopause?

The answer seems to be yes! An 8-week Pilates program for menopausal women was found to decrease hot flashes and night sweats. There were also improvements in psychological and physical symptoms. Flexibility and strength improved as well.[74] All that in 8 weeks.

TAI CHI

Tai Chi is an ancient, gentle mind-body practice that focuses on breathing and slow, deliberate movement (the flow). It has numerous health benefits including improved sleep, reducing symptoms of depression, anxiety and stress. It has also been shown to improve physical strength, balance and flexibility in women. It has even been shown to increase bone strength and improve lipid profiles.[75,76] But wait, there's more! For women in menopause, tai chi may be helpful in improving a range of symptoms and lowering risks for disease. Studies show tai chi may have a protective effect on metabolic and cardiovascular health, helping to reduce the risk of insulin resistance, lowering inflammation and improving cardiovascular function.[77]

As you can see, the connection between mind and body is a strong one. When you make that connection, you are on your way to better health and better mental health. We can all use a little more of that especially when menopause is making a mess of things.

Try out a couple of these techniques. When you find "the one," you'll know it.

MEDITATION, YOGA, PILATES AND OTHER WAYS TO TRANSFORM BODY AND SPIRIT

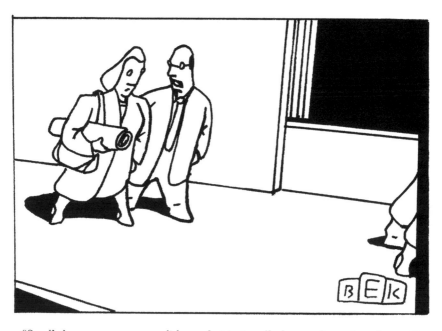

"So all these years you never did yoga but just walked around carrying the mat?"

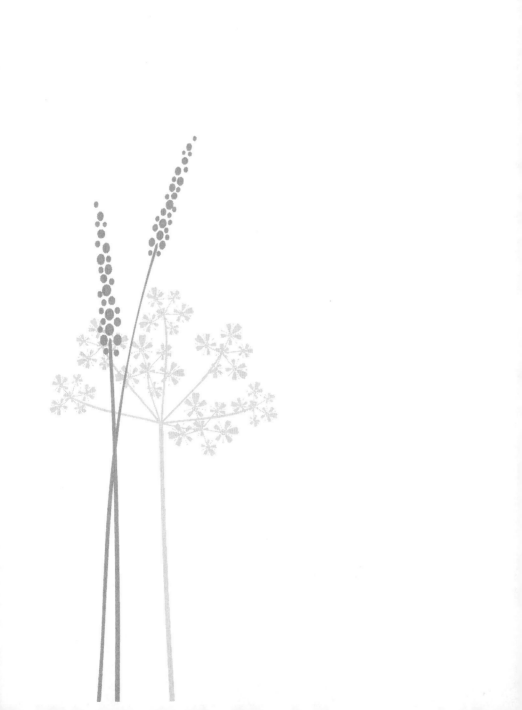

CHAPTER SEVENTEEN

Let's Talk Supplements

"I'm interested in women's health because I'm a woman. I'd be a darn fool not to be on my own side."

MAYA ANGELOU

As you go through menopause, your body is in a constant state of change. Systems are changing and adapting to what will be the new normal. This kind of change can put tremendous stress on your body. And when we're stressed, we draw a lot more on our reserves.

Good nutrition, of course, is vital to maintaining an optimal level of wellness. Ideally, we get our nutritional needs met through our diets. In theory, that's great. In practice, however, we often fall short of our goals. We don't always make the best food choices. (Hey, we're human.) And, in some cases, the quality of what we consume is just not optimal. In other cases, our bodies, for whatever reason, can't seem to get enough of some vital nutrient.

Whatever the reason, there are circumstances in which supplementation is helpful or even necessary. But is it as easy as running to the drug store and grabbing whatever multivitamin is on sale? Probably not.

So, let's talk about supplementation and what it means in the life of the menopausal woman.

THE GREAT SUPPLEMENT DEBATE

Supplementation, like any other issue, has its proponents and its critics. It has its reputable advocates and it has its snake oil vendors.

On the pro side, advocates for supplementation argue that menopausal and post-menopausal women are often lacking in key vitamins and minerals that are necessary for optimum health and wellness. Vitamin D, calcium, iron, vitamin K and others are frequently mentioned. Women are often deficient in some of these key nutrients. Proponents also argue that you just can't eat enough of the natural sources to get your optimal dose. Some insist that you should only buy supplements from sustainable, natural sourced companies. (Read that as pricey). Others claim that generic, low cost supplements from the local store are just fine.

On the con side, some proponents insist that you really don't need supplements at all.

At least on the surface, the differing opinions sound legitimate, right? Well it depends on who is saying it. Is it a credentialed nutritionist or dietician? Or is it a "legitimate sounding" spokesperson for the latest secret "proprietary blend" touting vitamins and minerals that will instantly relieve those night sweats? Hmm…if it's so good for us why can I only buy it on late night TV for a week's wages?

Unless you have a degree in nutrition, you're probably scratching your head and wondering what the truth is. Do I need supplementation? Is that TV proprietary blend better because it's proprietary?

It's enough to make you crazy! So, we're going to take a deep dive into the truth about supplementation based on the facts. Not the infomercials. What kinds of vitamins and minerals might a menopausal woman need? And why?

THE BIG DOGS

There are a few vitamins and minerals that we know women tend to be deficient in even if they're not menopausal. Some are especially important for optimum wellness for a woman in menopause. Let's take a look and see what the science, not the guy on TV, says.

IRON – IT'S COMPLICATED

Generally speaking, women are more likely than men to be iron deficient or anemic. We can blame that at least in part to our menstrual cycles. Women also tend to have a lower amount of red blood cells than men. Combined, this can result in iron deficiency. You're thinking, "Easy fix. Supplements. Right?" Not so fast, there. Iron is one of those minerals that too little OR too much can be dangerous, and the margin is narrow. Supplementation is sometimes recommended during menopause but under medical supervision. Because it's complicated.

Menopausal women can be iron deficient. It is not uncommon, especially if their periods have not yet ceased completely. But, an interesting thing happens during perimenopause. As your periods become less frequent and as your estrogen drops, your iron levels tend to increase.[78] By the time you complete menopause, your iron needs drop dramatically. So you have to be super careful with iron. Current thinking is that iron supplementation may not be necessary for menopausal and post-menopausal women because the need is declining. Sources of iron from the diet are the focus in most cases.[79]

HONORABLE MENTIONS

There are a few other supplements that are often recommended. Their efficacy in menopausal support is unclear but they are worthy of mention.

VITAMIN D – CALCIUM'S BFF

Sometimes called the "sunshine vitamin," vitamin D is essential to bone renewal, cell growth and hormone balance. It is called the sunshine vitamin because your body makes vitamin D naturally when you're in the sun. As we age, our ability to absorb vitamin D decreases and deficiency is not uncommon. This decreased availability can increase the risk of bone loss because vitamin D is calcium's BFF. Calcium needs vitamin D to work optimally.

Aside from its bone-protecting benefits, higher serum levels of vitamin D in people age 50 and older are associated with better perceived quality of life, improved mobility and lower levels of depression and anxiety.[80] Interestingly, recommendations for vitamin D supplementation for post-menopausal women is mixed. The concerns seem to be focused on the increased risk of kidney stones and cardiovascular issues in older women who take calcium and vitamin D for bone health.[81] Of course, getting vitamin D from foods like eggs, wild salmon and dairy products is important, but sometimes supplementation is recommended.

So the verdict on vitamin D seems to be ok if you're deficient during your pre and perimenopausal years but post-menopause, the game changes. Because vitamin D is a powerhouse in the body (and sometimes referred to as having a hormone-like quality), supplementation should be done as part of your overall health plan with your healthcare provider. Always err on the side of caution. Your body will thank you.

CALCIUM – THE BONE BUILDER

Calcium is the building block for strong, healthy bones. Most of us have been told by our healthcare providers to take our calcium+D supplements, right? And there's good reason. As we enter menopause, the loss of estrogen can accelerate the rate of bone loss that we naturally experience. Maintaining adequate calcium stores helps us to balance out what we lose. The vitamin D is calcium's BFF and helps with the absorption and bioavailability of calcium in the body.

It is generally recommended that perimenopausal women maintain their calcium intake either through diet or through supplementation to protect bone health. Good sources of calcium include dairy products, dark green leafy vegetables, beans and peas, tofu, seeds, nuts and some fish. Some foods may be fortified with calcium, like orange juice, cereal and breakfast bars.[82]

For those who require supplementation, the National Institutes of Health[82] recommend:

- For pre-menopausal women 25-50 years old and post-menopausal women on estrogen replacement therapy: 1,000-1,200 milligrams of calcium per day.
- For post-menopausal women less than age 65 not on estrogen replacement therapy: 1,500 milligrams of calcium per day.

Your particular needs may be more or less depending on your health status. Always consult with your healthcare provider so that you are getting maximum benefit and minimizing risks.

VITAMIN K - THE NEW KID ON THE BLOCK

Vitamin K is a little known vitamin that is getting lots of attention especially in the areas of bone health and cardiovascular health, both concerns for women entering the menopause years. We have vitamin K in our bodies and use it, particularly the most bio-available form K2, for building bone. Vitamin K works with vitamin D which work with calcium to build and maintain strong bones. How that works is not well understood. Vitamin K is also being recognized as a key player in cardiovascular health and insulin sensitivity.[83]

What we know about vitamin K is that as our estrogen declines, it gets harder to absorb and use vitamin K. Deficiency is not uncommon. Dietary sources include high-fat dairy products from grass-fed cows, egg yolks, as well as liver and other organ meats, fermented foods like sauerkraut and miso. If you choose to supplement, K2 supplements are available. K2 may be most effective when combined with vitamin D because of their synergistic relationship.[84,85]

VITAMIN E - OLD SCHOOL HELP

Vitamin E was once the darling of the vitamin world. Over the years, it has been overshadowed by the new kids. But, there was a time when vitamin E was commonly used to treat hot flashes. Unfortunately the research is extremely limited. The studies that were done seem to support the claims that vitamin E is effective in decreasing the frequency and intensity of hot flashes.[86,87]

So there you have it, the 411 on the supplements that may be helpful in managing your journey through menopause more comfortably and healthful.

As always, before you decide to supplement, talk with your healthcare provider. Vitamins and minerals are not benign and can have powerful effects in the body, not to mention interactions with other drugs you may be taking. Remember, just because it's over the counter does not mean it is right for you. And, more is not always better. Better is better.

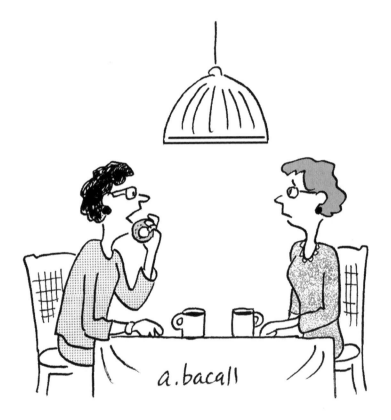

"I'm really not eating a balanced diet. I'm always replacing meals with snacks. Maybe I should be taking a multivitamin before I eat a donut."

WHERE MENOPAUSE MEETS CULTURE

"You can be a thousand different women. It's your choice which one you want to be. It's about freedom and sovereignty. You celebrate who you are. You say, 'This is my kingdom.'"

Salma Hayek

In previous chapters, we've seen that throughout history, women experiencing menopause have been treated differently. Sometimes treated rather badly. Thankfully, attitudes have changed over time and no one thinks we're witches anymore…well, not real witches anyway.

Let's put external perceptions aside for a minute and talk about menopause from OUR perspective – as women. Given that menopause is a universal experience for women, it is tempting to think that we all experience it in the same ways. After all, we all undergo the biologically-driven changes that result in cessation of menses. But how do we experience menopause? Is it the same for all of us?

Research says no, we don't. And it goes beyond individual differences. If we're all women going through "the change," then what's going on? The answer lies in the foundations of culture.

The fact is, when we talk about the experience of menopause, we're talking about more than just the biological changes that occur. Our menopause occurs within the larger context in which we live our lives. So, we have to consider not only the biological changes, but we also have to consider where and how the experience occurs. That "where and how" is driven in large part by our respective social and cultural foundations.

WHAT DOES CULTURE HAVE TO DO WITH MENOPAUSE?

More than you might think.

Culture is more than just your neighborhood or your nationality. It is more than just race or ethnicity or religion. It is all those things and more. There are a lot of definitions of culture but essentially, culture is generally defined as the knowledge, beliefs and customs that are created by a group of people for perceiving, interpreting, understanding and responding to the world around them.

Put another way, who we are and where we come from influences how we interpret and operate in the world. For example, what one group of people (culture) may see as adversity, another group may see the same situation as a blessing. Our unique cultural experiences are what account for the different ways people handle disasters and bountiful harvests and births and deaths and every event of life – and yes, even menopause.

In large part, we believe what we are taught to believe. As such, when faced with a situation, we not only have the actual experience, we also interpret that experience through the framework of values, beliefs and such that we've learned.

Think about this: Remember when you were a child and went to the doctor knowing you were going to get a shot? Scary for most kids, right? You just KNEW it was going to hurt. So, you were already expecting the pain before you even got there. What happened when the doctor walked in? The needle wasn't even out yet and you were probably crying. And, before the stick even happened, you might have been crying that it hurt. Before. The. Stick. Even. Happened.

Did it really hurt? Maybe at the actual moment of the stick. But, the brain and its anticipation were primed for pain before anything even happened. This is actually a common scenario and this anticipation of pain or discomfort is what triggers the reaction.

A really smart neurologist, V. S. Ramachandran, actually describes this pain phenomenon in this way: pain is an opinion. In the simplest terms, the brain decides there is or will be pain (even if there is NO pain or injury), and we can experience pain. The fear of pain can make minor pain worse. The opposite is also true. A person can experience pain or an injury of some kind and experience less pain than might be expected especially when they are not worried about discomfort or are not fully aware of the extent of an injury.[90] It's all about how we perceive something.

So what does this brain thing have to do with culture and menopause? Everything. We are raised to be fearful of certain things, to expect certain things and even to embrace certain things. How your culture deals with menopause will influence how you think about and experience menopause.

MENOPAUSE ACROSS CULTURES

Of all the individual differences that we know women experience during menopause, there are also differences in the way women of different cultures experience menopause. It is not a one-size-fits-all experience by any means. And, researchers have taken notice.

Let's take a quick trip around the world:

- In one of the earliest studies of menopause and culture, Indian women of the Rajput caste in India reported few, if any, issues with menopausal symptoms other than changes in their cycle.[91] More recent studies have found that, when women do report symptoms, there is a distinct difference in the menopausal experience between women in rural and urban areas.[92]
- In Australia, researchers found that the perception of and experience of menopause was significantly different for indigenous vs. non-indigenous women. In the Indigenous culture, elders are respected, and menopause is associated with a gain in status or prestige.[93] Another study found that "menopause" was not a common term used within the culture and that women likely didn't associate symptoms with a cessation of menses.[94]
- Women in Islamic and many African societies report fewer symptoms of menopause which is thought to be influenced in part by the relaxation of certain gender roles post-menopause.[95]
- Among Turkish women, the views of menopause were mixed. Over 90% viewed the cessation of menses negatively and representative of the "loss of youth." A majority also viewed menopause as positive due to the end of pregnancy risk and dealing with periods.[96]

- Native American women tend to view menopause as a neutral or positive experience. Post-menopausal women are considered sages within their communities and hold a high level of status.[98] They don't even have a word for menopause.
- Women in Asian cultures tend to report very few menopausal symptoms. When they do, the most common symptom reported is hot flashes. Interestingly, the Japanese have a word for this time of a woman's reproductive life – konenki. Literally translated, ko means "renewal and regeneration," nen means "year" or "years" and ki means "season" or "energy." In Japanese culture, konenki is used to describe a gradual transition to the next phase of life. In fact, until very recently, the Japanese didn't even have a word for hot flash![99]
- Women in western cultures tend to view menopause more negatively. It is often seen as a loss of youth, a loss of fertility and even womanhood. Symptoms tend to be frequently reported and viewed in a medical context to be "treated."[93]
- Mayan women in Mexico generally report no significant menopausal symptoms other than the cessation of their cycles. One hypothesis for this phenomenon speculates that because child-bearing is a significant part of their adult lives, they remain in a constant state of relatively low estrogen. Thus, when menopause occurs, the biochemical impacts may be less intense.[95]

There are many more examples of how menopause is viewed across cultures. And this is all fine and good to know, right? You never know when you might need some good menopause trivia. Seriously, these differences are important because who we are and where we're from matters.

HOW DOES YOUR CULTURAL BACKGROUND AFFECT YOUR EXPERIENCE OF MENOPAUSE?

Not unexpectedly, a woman's ethnicity or race also seems to impact their experience of menopause and its health impacts. This is especially true for women of color.

MENOPAUSE CONSIDERATIONS FOR WOMEN OF COLOR

"We delight in the beauty of the butterfly, but rarely admit the changes it has gone through to achieve that beauty."
MAYA ANGELOU

When you look at the different ways culture influences the experience of menopause, women in many cultures seem to not experience menopause in the negative, distressing ways others do. In fact, women in western cultures seem to really struggle with the negative symptoms of menopause and frequently seek medical intervention.[98]

If you fall into one of those groups that seem to have a pretty easy go with menopausal symptoms, you might be tempted to think, "Yay, a few hot flashes and missed periods and I'm done." Not so fast. The fact is, menopause is more than just the cessation of your period.

Menopause is a process that results in significant long-term changes in your body. And, along with those changes come health risks. Your two primary female sex hormones, estrogen and progesterone, start declining as your body begins to shut down its reproductive capabilities. These hormones, especially estrogen, are linked to bodily functions separate and apart from reproduction. As we've discussed in previous chapters, estrogen plays a key role in maintaining heart health, bone health, breast health, brain health and more. For women of color, some of these health impacts seem to be more significant and, in some cases, more severe. This doesn't mean that you're destined to have these struggles. It does mean that you need to know your risks and take action to mitigate those risks where you can.

HEART HEALTH

It is well-documented in the literature that following menopause, a woman's risk of heart disease increases significantly. Estrogen has a protective effect for women and prior to mid-life, a woman's risk of heart disease is relatively low. As estrogen declines, a woman's risk for heart disease dramatically increases. In fact, cardiovascular disease (CVD) is the number one cause of death in American women, claiming over 400,000 lives each year, or one death every 80 seconds.[99] That's more than cancer, respiratory disease and diabetes combined.

For women of color, the risk of heart disease and death from heart disease is even higher. Here are some facts that might surprise you:

- The occurrence of cardiovascular disease among African American women is about 45% compared to about 35% for Caucasian women.[100]
- The death rate from CVD is 15% higher for African American women compared to other groups.[100]
- About a third of Mexican American women have cardiovascular disease.[100]
- South Asian (Indian) women get heart disease earlier, have higher rates of heart disease and die from more often from heart problems when compared to other Asian groups and Caucasians.[101]

Interestingly, women from other Asian groups (Japanese, Vietnamese, etc.) have historically had a lower incidence of cardiovascular disease than other groups. However, according to a United Nations report, the risk of CVD in the Asian population has been gradually increasing as lifestyles are changing and becoming more sedentary and "westernized." This change has been specifically noted in Asians who move to North America.[102]

Another important factor that contributes to the increased risk of CVD for women of color seems to point to lifestyle. Women of color tend to have more risk factors for CVD[100] including:

- Higher cholesterol levels
- Obesity
- Diabetes

- Diets high in saturated and trans fats
- Smoking
- Physical inactivity
- Uncontrolled high blood pressure

So what can you do? The American Heart Association encourages women to take control of their health and know your numbers!

- See your doctor regularly.
- Get your cholesterol, blood pressure, weight and blood sugar checked regularly.
- Increase physical activity
- If you smoke, stop.
- Eat a healthy diet.

BREAST HEALTH

As we've discussed in previous chapters, breast cancer is not thought to be directly related to menopause. However, breast cancer risk tends to increase with age and coincides with the time when women are experiencing menopause.

For women of color and certain ethnicities, there seems to be some correlation between breast cancer and the process of menopause. In a long-term study known as the Multiethnic Cohort Study, Native Hawaiians were found to have the highest incidence of postmenopausal breast cancer. African American women and Latinas had much lower rates. Asian and White women fell somewhere in between.[102]

For South Asian women (women from India), breast cancer is of particular concern. Rates are increasing with breast cancer now accounting for 25% to 32% of all female cancers reported in India. Researchers are also finding a trend towards earlier onset of breast cancer among this group. While most cases are found in women over the age of 50, an increasing number of Indian women are being diagnosed before age 50.[103] It isn't clear why this trend is occurring but there is some research to suggest that the traditional Indian diet and changes in lifestyle may be affecting health.[104]

So what's the takeaway here? Protect the girls. Know your risks. Do your self-exams and get your mammograms as recommended by your healthcare provider.

Exactly why these differences between cultures and ethnicities occur is unclear. It is suspected that the differences may be due in part to differing levels of hormones in the body. Diet, lifestyle – even genetics – seem to be key players. There is just so much we don't know yet.

In the meantime, you can be proactive about your health.

- Watch your diet
- Get some exercise
- Don't smoke
- If you're overweight, losing even 5% of your body weight can have huge benefits
- Know your risks
- Know your numbers – have your cholesterol, blood pressure, weight, glucose and other important measures checked regularly
- Get your mammograms and bone density screens
- If you experience ANY concerns, see your healthcare provider sooner rather than later

Menopause doesn't have to mean declining health. Do your best to live a healthy lifestyle and work with a healthcare provider you trust. Together you can make the choices that are right for your needs.

CONCLUSION

"So many women I've talked to see menopause as an ending. But I've discovered this is your moment to reinvent yourself after years of focusing on the needs of everyone else. It's your opportunity to get clear about what matters to you and then to pursue that with all of your energy, time and talent."

Oprah Winfrey

So, my friend, here we are at the end of our time together. We've talked about a lot of things, some of them quite personal. Hopefully, you've found some answers that you've been seeking and learned some things that will carry you through your journey.

As you go along, there will be days of great joy, of frustration and maybe even some sadness. Allow yourself to fully experience them all. These experiences will each leave you with a nugget of wisdom that you will carry forever. You can never have too many nuggets.

The transition through menopause is a challenge and a time of self-reflection as you prepare for a new beginning. You are embarking on the next phase of your life. Where do you want to go? Who will you be?

Dare to dream!

Be well and step boldly into your future.

"I think the best role models for women are people who are fruitfully and confidently themselves, who bring light into the world."

Meryl Streep

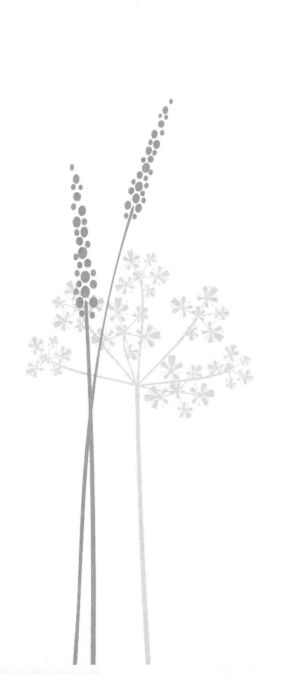

ABOUT DR. SOMA MANDAL

MIDLIFE WOMEN'S HEALTH & MENOPAUSE SPECIALIST

Widely regarded as one of America's top physicians in midlife women's health, Dr. Soma Mandal is a board-certified internist who has helped thousands of women to successfully navigate menopause and reinvent themselves along the way. Earning her MD at New York University School of Medicine, and a prestigious research fellowship at Oxford University in England, Dr. Mandal brings a fresh perspective to the topic of menopause, particularly for women of color.

Fusing traditional Western medicine with her Eastern roots, Dr. Mandal's approach combines the best of both worlds. Her unique approach provides women with a much-needed, easy-to follow process, making the forties and fifties plus, *fabulous*.

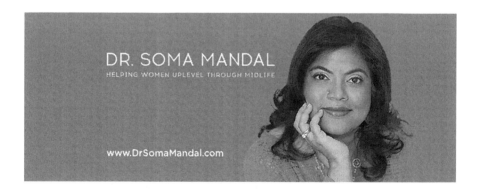

CONTACT DR. SOMA MANDAL

Dr. Soma Mandal would love to hear from you!

You can get in touch with her by connecting with her on Facebook and Twitter or visiting her website at **www.DrSomaMandal.com**.

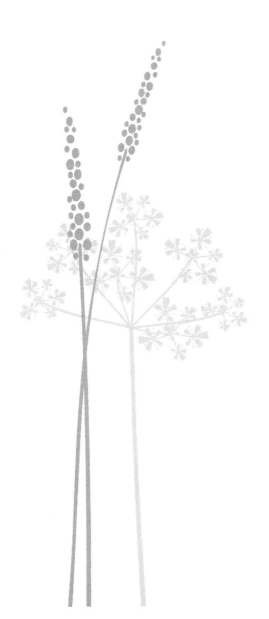

REFERENCES

[1] Parkin, T. G. (2004). Old Age in the Roman World: A Cultural and Social History. Johns Hopkins University Press.

[2] Sweeney, D. (n.d.). Elder Women in Ancient Egypt. Retrieved from http://archaeology.tau.ac.il/elder-women-in-ancient-egypt

[3] Hildegard, S. (2006). Causes and Cures: The Complete English Translation of Hildegardis Causae Et Curae Libri V.

[4] Mulder-Bakker, A. B., & Nip, R. (2004). The Prime of Their Lives: Wise Old Women in Pre-industrial Europe. Peeters Pub & Booksellers.

[5] Monter, W. (1987). Protestant Wives, Catholic Saints, and the Devil's handmaid: Women in the Age of the Reformations. In Becoming Visible: Women in European History Bridenthal, R., Koonz, C., Stuard, S. M. (eds).

[6] Baron, Y. M. (2012). A History of the Menopause. The Department of Obstetrics and Gynaecology, University of Malta.

[7] Rosenhek, J. (2014, February). Mad with menopause. Retrieved from http://www.doctorsreview.com/history/mad-menopause/

[8] Simoni, R. D., Hill, R. L., & Vaughn, M. (2002). The Discovery of Estrone, Estriol, and Estradiol and the Biochemical Study of Reproduction. The Work of Edward Adelbert Doisy. The Journal of Biological Chemistry, 277(28), 35-36.

[9] Matthews, K. A. (1992). Myths and realities of the menopause. Psychosomatic Medicine, 54(1), 1-9.

[10] Sarrel, P. M., Sullivan, S. D., & Nelson, L. M. (2016). Hormone replacement therapy in young women with surgical primary ovarian insufficiency. Fertility and sterility, 106(7), 1580–1587.

[11] Morrow, P. K., Mattair, D. N., & Hortobagyi, G. N. (2011). Hot flashes: a review of pathophysiology and treatment modalities. The oncologist, 16(11), 1658–1664.

[12] How Do I Know I'm in Menopause? | The North American Menopause Society, NAMS. (n.d.). Retrieved from https://www.menopause.org/for-women/menopauseflashes/menopause-symptoms-and-treatments/how-do-i-know-i%27m-in-menopause-

[13] Hormone Level Tests. (n.d.). Retrieved from https://www.earlymenopause.com/information/tests/

[14] Anti-Müllerian Hormone Test. (n.d.). Retrieved from https://medlineplus.gov/lab-tests/anti-mullerian-hormone-test/

[15] Perimenopause, Early Menopause Symptoms | The North American Menopause Society, NAMS. (n.d.). Retrieved from https://www.menopause.org/for-women/menopauseflashes/menopause-symptoms-and-treatments/menopause-101-a-primer-for-the-perimenopausal

16. Kumar, A. B., Shamim, H., & Nagaraju, U. (2018). Premature Graying of Hair: Review with Updates. International journal of trichology, 10(5), 198–203. doi:10.4103/ijt.ijt_47_18
17. Ramos, P. M., & Miot, H. A. (2015). Female Pattern Hair Loss: a clinical and pathophysiological review. Anais brasileiros de dermatologia, 90(4), 529–543.
18. Brough, K. R., & Torgerson, R. R. (2017). Hormonal therapy in female pattern hair loss. International journal of women's dermatology, 3(1), 53–57.
19. Zarei, M., Wikramanayake, T. C., Falto-Aizpurua, L., Schachner, L. A., & Jimenez, J. J. (2016). Low level laser therapy and hair regrowth: an evidence-based review. Lasers in Medical Science, 31(2), 363-371.
20. Zárate, S., Stevnsner, T., & Gredilla, R. (2017). Role of Estrogen and Other Sex Hormones in Brain Aging. Neuroprotection and DNA Repair. Frontiers in aging neuroscience, 9, 430.
21. Derbyshire E. (2018). Brain Health across the Lifespan: A Systematic Review on the Role of Omega-3 Fatty Acid Supplements. Nutrients, 10(8), 1094.
22. Mohammady, M., Janani, L., Jahanfar, S., & Mousavi, M. S. (2018). Effect of omega-3 supplements on vasomotor symptoms in menopausal women: A systematic review and meta-analysis. European Journal of Obstetrics & Gynecology and Reproductive Biology, 228, 295-302.
23. Mandolesi, L., Polverino, A., Montuori, S., Foti, F., Ferraioli, G., Sorrentino, P., & Sorrentino, G. (2018). Effects of Physical Exercise on Cognitive Functioning and Wellbeing: Biological and Psychological Benefits. Frontiers in psychology, 9, 509.
24. Kataria, K., Dhar, A., Srivastava, A., Kumar, S., & Goyal, A. (2014). A systematic review of current understanding and management of mastalgia. The Indian journal of surgery, 76(3), 217–222.
25. Lee, I. (2003). Physical Activity and Cancer Prevention???Data from Epidemiologic Studies. Medicine & Science in Sports & Exercise, 35(11), 1823-1827.
26. Brown, K. (2017, March 6). Breast Self-Exam Guidelines: Johns Hopkins Breast Center. Retrieved from https://www.hopkinsmedicine.org/breast_center/treatments_services/breast_cancer_screening/breast_self_exam.html
27. NBCF. (n.d.). Breast Self-Exam :: The National Breast Cancer Foundation. Retrieved from https://www.nationalbreastcancer.org/breast-self-exam
28. NBCF. (n.d.). Mammogram :: The National Breast Cancer Foundation. Retrieved from https://www.nationalbreastcancer.org/mammogram
29. What Is Breast Cancer Screening? (2018, December 17). Retrieved from https://www.cdc.gov/cancer/breast/basic_info/screening.htm
30. Menopause and Heart Disease. (n.d.). Retrieved from https://www.heart.org/en/health-topics/consumer-healthcare/menopause-and-heart-disease
31. Iorga, A., Cunningham, C. M., Moazeni, S., Ruffenach, G., Umar, S., & Eghbali, M. (2017). The protective role of estrogen and estrogen receptors in cardiovascular disease and the controversial use of estrogen therapy. Biology of sex differences, 8(1), 3.

REFERENCES

32. 2019 ACC/AHA Guideline on the Primary Prevention of Cardiovascular Disease. (2019). Retrieved from https://www.ahajournals.org/doi/10.1161/CIR.0000000000000678
33. Flint, A. J., Rexrode, K. M., Hu, F. B., Glynn, R. J., Caspard, H., Manson, J. E., … Rimm, E. B. (2010). Body mass index, waist circumference, and risk of coronary heart disease: A prospective study among men and women. Obesity Research & Clinical Practice, 4(3), e171-e181.
34. Kromhout, D., Menotti, A., Kesteloot, H., & Sans, S. (2002). Prevention of Coronary Heart Disease by Diet and Lifestyle. Circulation, 105(7), 893-898.
35. Dalen, J. E., & Devries, S. (2014). Diets to Prevent Coronary Heart Disease 1957-2013: What Have We Learned? The American Journal of Medicine, 127(5), 364-369.
36. Preventing Heart Disease. (2019, January 30). Retrieved from https://www.hsph.harvard.edu/nutritionsource/disease-prevention/cardiovascular-disease/preventing-cvd/
37. The American Heart Association Diet and Lifestyle Recommendations. (n.d.). Retrieved from https://www.heart.org/en/healthy-living/healthy-eating/eat-smart/nutrition-basics/aha-diet-and-lifestyle-recommendations
38. Smoking and Your Heart. (n.d.). Retrieved from https://www.nhlbi.nih.gov/health-topics/smoking-and-your-heart
39. Prior, J. C. (2014, June 19). Perimenopause and Thyroid Problems:common and confusing. Retrieved from https://www.cemcor.ubc.ca/ask/perimenopause-and-thyroid-problems-common-and-confusing
40. Davis, S. R., Castelo-Branco, C., Chedraui, P., Lumsden, M. A., Nappi, R. E., & Shah, D. (2012). Understanding weight gain at menopause. Climacteric, 15(5), 419-429.
41. Koutras, D. A. (1997). Disturbances of Menstruation in Thyroid Disease. Annals of the New York Academy of Sciences, 816(1 Adolescent Gy), 280-284.
42. Perimenopausal Bleeding and Bleeding After Menopause. (n.d.). Retrieved from https://www.acog.org/Patients/FAQs/Perimenopausal-Bleeding-and-Bleeding-After-Menopause?
43. Caring for your skin in menopause. (n.d.). Retrieved from https://www.aad.org/public/skin-hair-nails/skin-care/skin-care-during-menopause
44. The True Effects Of Menopause. (2012, May 31). Retrieved from https://www.americannursetoday.com/blog/the-true-effects-of-menopause/
45. Palacios S, Nappi RE, Bruyniks N, et al. The European Vulvovaginal Epidemiological Survey (EVES): prevalence, symptoms and impact of vulvovaginal atrophy of menopause. Climacteric. 2018;21(3):286–291.
46. Cosmetic Procedures. (n.d.). Retrieved from https://www.plasticsurgery.org/cosmetic-procedures
47. Statement from FDA Commissioner Scott Gottlieb, M.D., on efforts to safeguard women's health from deceptive health claims and significant risks related to devices marketed for use in medical procedures for 'vaginal rejuvenation? (2018, August 2). Retrieved from https://www.fda.gov/news-events/press-announcements/statement-fda-commissioner-scott-gottlieb-md-efforts-safeguard-womens-health-deceptive-health-claims

48. Kronenberg, F. (1990). Hot Flashes: Epidemiology and Physiologya. Annals of the New York Academy of Sciences, 592(1), 52-86.
49. Feldman, B. M., Voda, A., & Gronseth, E. (1985). The prevalence of hot flash and associated variables among perimenopausal women. Research in Nursing & Health, 8(3), 261-268.
50. Menopause and your bone health. (2018, April 26). Retrieved from https://www.nhs.uk/live-well/healthy-body/menopause-and-your-bone-health/
51. Osteoporosis and Low Bone Mass - What Is the Difference and What Can I Do? (2015, February). Retrieved from https://www.health.ny.gov/publications/1986/index.htm
52. Santos, L., Elliott-Sale, K. J., & Sale, C. (2017). Exercise and bone health across the lifespan. Biogerontology, 18(6), 931–946.
53. Wippert, P. M., Rector, M., Kuhn, G., & Wuertz-Kozak, K. (2017). Stress and Alterations in Bones: An Interdisciplinary Perspective. Frontiers in endocrinology, 8, 96.
54. Menopause & Osteoporosis. (n.d.). Retrieved from https://my.clevelandclinic.org/health/articles/10091-menopause--osteoporosis
55. The NAMS 2017 Hormone Therapy Position Statement Advisory Panel. The 2017 hormone therapy position statement of the North American Menopause Society. Menopause. 2017;24(7):728-753.
56. ACOG Practice Bulletin No. 141: management of menopausal symptoms. Obstet Gynecol. 2014;123(1):202-216.
57. Stuenkel CA, Davis SR, Gompel A, et al. Treatment of symptoms of the menopause: an Endocrine Society Clinical Practice Guideline. J Clin Endocrinol Metab. 2015;100(11):3975-4011.
58. Women's Health Concern, 'Complementary/alternative therapies for menopausal women', (2017). https://www.womens-health-concern.org/help-and-advice/factsheets/complementaryalternative-therapies-menopausal-women/
59. National Institute for Health and Care Excellence. (2015, February 10). Complementary/alternative therapies for menopausal women. Retrieved from https://www.womens-health-concern.org/help-and-advice/factsheets/complementaryalternative-therapies-menopausal-women/
60. Lund KS, Siersma V, Brodersen J, et al. (2019). Efficacy of a standardized acupuncture approach for women with bothersome menopausal symptoms: a pragmatic randomized study in primary care (the ACOM study.) BMJ Open 9:e023637.
61. Mann, E., Smith, M. J., Hellier, J., Balabanovic, J. A., Hamed, H., Grunfeld, E. A., & Hunter, M. S. (2012). Cognitive behavioural treatment for women who have menopausal symptoms after breast cancer treatment (MENOS 1): a randomised controlled trial. The Lancet. Oncology, 13(3), 309–318.
62. Wijma, K., Melin, A., Nedstrand, E., & Hammar, M. (1997). Treatment of menopausal symptoms with applied relaxation: A pilot study. Journal of Behavior Therapy and Experimental Psychiatry, 28(4), 251-261.

REFERENCES

63. Traditional Chinese Medicine for Natural Menopause Relief. (2019, February 21). Retrieved from https://www.pacificcollege.edu/news/blog/2015/01/30/traditional-chinese-medicine-natural-menopause-relief

64. Zhu, X., Liew, Y., & Liu, Z. L. (2016). Chinese herbal medicine for menopausal symptoms. The Cochrane database of systematic reviews, 3, CD009023.

65. Yang, H., Yang, J., Wen, Z., Zha, Q., Nie, G., Huang, X., ... Wang, X. (2012). Effect of combining therapy with traditional chinese medicine-based psychotherapy and herbal medicines in women with menopausal syndrome: a randomized controlled clinical trial. Evidence-based complementary and alternative medicine : eCAM, 2012, 354145.

66. Black Cohosh. (2016, November 29). Retrieved from https://nccih.nih.gov/health/blackcohosh/ataglance.htm

67. Abdali, K., Khajehei, M., & Tabatabaee, H. R. (2010). Effect of St John's wort on severity, frequency, and duration of hot flashes in premenopausal, perimenopausal and postmenopausal women. Menopause, 17(2), 326-331.

68. The History of Hypnosis. (n.d.). Retrieved from http://www.historyofhypnosis.org/

69. Elkins GR, Fisher WI, Johnson AK, et al. Clinical hypnosis in the treatment of postmenopausal hot flashes: a randomized controlled trial. Menopause. 2013;20(3):291–298.

70. Sood R, Kuhle CL, Kapoor E, Thielen JM, Frohmader KS, Mara KC, Faubion SS.(2019) Association of mindfulness and stress with menopausal symptoms in midlife women. Climacteric. 22 (4):377-382 Epub 2019 Jan 17

71. Innes, K. E., Selfe, T. K., & Vishnu, A. (2010). Mind-body therapies for menopausal symptoms: a systematic review. Maturitas, 66(2), 135–149.

72. Wong, C., Yip, B. H., Gao, T., Lam, K., Woo, D., Yip, A., ... Wong, S. (2018). Mindfulness-Based Stress Reduction (MBSR) or Psychoeducation for the Reduction of Menopausal Symptoms: A Randomized, Controlled Clinical Trial. Scientific reports, 8(1), 6609.

73. Carmody, J. F., Crawford, S., Salmoirago-Blotcher, E., Leung, K., Churchill, L., & Olendzki, N. (2011). Mindfulness training for coping with hot flashes: results of a randomized trial. Menopause (New York, N.Y.), 18(6), 611–620.

74. Lee, H., Caguicla, J. M., Park, S., Kwak, D. J., Won, D. Y., Park, Y., ... Kim, M. (2016). Effects of 8-week Pilates exercise program on menopausal symptoms and lumbar strength and flexibility in postmenopausal women. Journal of exercise rehabilitation, 12(3), 247–251.

75. Wen, J., & Kang, Y. (2004). The Effects Of Taichi On Bone Mineral Density And Lipid Profiles In Postmenopausal Women. Medicine & Science in Sports & Exercise, 36(Supplement), S58.

76. Sun, Z., Chen, H., Berger, M. R., Zhang, L., Guo, H., & Huang, Y. (2016). Effects of tai chi exercise on bone health in perimenopausal and postmenopausal women: a systematic review and meta-analysis. Osteoporosis International, 27(10), 2901-2911.

77. Siu, P. M., Yu, A. P., Yu, D. S., Hui, S. S., & Woo, J. (2017). Effectiveness of Tai Chi training to alleviate metabolic syndrome in abdominal obese older adults: a randomised controlled trial. The Lancet, 390, S11.

78. Jian, J., Pelle, E., & Huang, X. (2009). Iron and menopause: does increased iron affect the health of postmenopausal women?. Antioxidants & redox signaling, 11(12), 2939–2943.

79. Iron Supplementation Typically Not Recommended for Postmenopausal Women. (2011, September 9). Retrieved from https://newsnetwork.mayoclinic.org/discussion/iron-supplementation-typically-not-recommended-for-postmenopausal-women/

80. Milart, P., Woźniakowska, E., & Wrona, W. (2018). Selected vitamins and quality of life in menopausal women. Przegląd menopauzalny = Menopause review, 17(4), 175–179.

81. Aggarwal, S., & Nityanand (2013). Calcium and vitamin D in post menopausal women. Indian journal of endocrinology and metabolism, 17(Suppl 3), S618–S620.

82. Calcium. (2018, September 26). Retrieved from https://ods.od.nih.gov/factsheets/Calcium-HealthProfessional/

83. DiNicolantonio, J. J., Bhutani, J., & O'Keefe, J. H. (2015). The health benefits of vitamin K. Open heart, 2(1), e000300.

84. Leech, J. (2018, September 21). Vitamin K2: Everything You Need to Know. Retrieved from https://www.healthline.com/nutrition/vitamin-k2#sources

85. Kidd, P. M. (2010). Vitamins D and K as pleiotropic nutrients: clinical importance to the skeletal and cardiovascular systems and preliminary evidence for synergy. Alternative Medicine Review, 15(3), 199-222.

86. Ziaei, S., Kazemnejad, A., & Zareai, M. (2007). The Effect of Vitamin E on Hot Flashes in Menopausal Women. Gynecologic and Obstetric Investigation, 64(4), 204-207.

87. Philp HA. (2003). Hot flashes: a review of the literature on alternative and complementary treatment approaches. Alter Med Rev, 8, 284–302.

88. Ramachandran, V. S. (1999). Phantoms in the Brain: Probing the Mysteries of the Human Mind. New York, NY: HarperCollins.

89. Flint, M. (1975). The menopause: Reward or punishment? Psychosomatics: Journal of Consultation and Liaison Psychiatry, 16(4), 161-163.

90. Unni J. (2010). Third consensus meeting of Indian Menopause Society (2008): A summary. Journal of mid-life health, 1(1), 43–47.

91. Jones, E. K., Jurgenson, J. R., Katzenellenbogen, J. M., & Thompson, S. C. (2012). Menopause and the influence of culture: another gap for Indigenous Australian women?. BMC women's health, 12, 43.

92. Davis, S. R., Knight, S., White, V., Claridge, C., Davis, B. J., & Bell, R. (2003). Climacteric symptoms among indigenous Australian women and a model for the use of culturally relevant art in health promotion. Menopause, 10(4), 345-351.

93. Beyene, Y. (1986). Cultural significance and physiological manifestations of menopause a biocultural analysis. Culture, Medicine and Psychiatry, 10(1), 47-71.

94. Ayranci, U., Orsal, O., Orsal, O., Arslan, G., & Emeksiz, D. F. (2010). Menopause status and attitudes in a Turkish midlife female population: an epidemiological study. BMC women's health, 10, 1.

95. Madden, S., St Pierre-Hansen, N., Kelly, L., Cromarty, H., Linkewich, B., & Payne, L. (2010). First Nations women's knowledge of menopause: experiences and perspectives. Canadian family physician Medecin de famille canadien, 56(9), e331–e337.

96. Melby, M. K. (2005). Factor analysis of climacteric symptoms in Japan. Maturitas, 52(3-4), 205-222.

97. Lock, M. (2002). Symptom reporting at menopause: a review of cross-cultural findings. British Menopause Society Journal, 8(4), 132-136.

98. Benjamin, EJ., et al. (2018). Heart Disease and Stroke Statistics-2018 Update: A Report From the American Heart Association.

99. American Heart Association. (2014). FACTS: Cardiovascular Disease: Women's No. 1 Health Threat. Retrieved from FACTS Cardiovascular Disease: Women's No. 1 Health Threatpublic/@wcm/@adv/documents/downloadable/ucm_462778.pdf

100. Atherosclerotic Cardiovascular Disease in South Asians in the United States: Epidemiology, Risk Factors, and Treatments: A Scientific Statement From the American Heart Association. (3, July). Retrieved from https://ahajournals.org/doi/10.1161/CIR.0000000000000580

101. Reinhardt, E. (2005). The Atlas of heart disease and stroke. UN Chronicle, 42(1).

102. University of Hawaii Cancer Center. (n.d.). Multiethnic Cohort (MEC) Study. Retrieved from https://www.uhcancercenter.org/mec

103. Shah, S. (n.d.). Trends of Breast Cancer in India. Retrieved from http://www.breastcancerindia.net/statistics/trends.html

104. Sinha R., Anderson D., McDonald S., Greenwald P. (2003). Cancer risk and diet in India. Journal of Postgraduate Medicine, 49(3), 222–228.

Made in the
USA
Lexington, KY

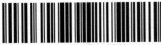